Critical Pedagogy in

19959174

Sue Dyson

Critical Pedagogy in Nursing

Transformational Approaches to Nurse Education in a Globalized World

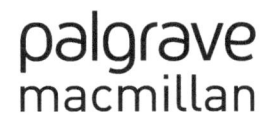

palgrave
macmillan

Sue Dyson
School of Health and Education
Middlesex University
London, UK

ISBN 978-1-349-84932-1   ISBN 978-1-137-56891-5 (eBook)
DOI 10.1057/978-1-137-56891-5

Library of Congress Control Number: 2017947188

© The Editor(s) (if applicable) and The Author(s) 2018
Softcover reprint of the hardcover 1st edition 2018 978-1-137-56890-8
The author(s) has/have asserted their right(s) to be identified as the author(s) of this work in accordance with the Copyright, Designs and Patents Act 1988.
This work is subject to copyright. All rights are solely and exclusively licensed by the Publisher, whether the whole or part of the material is concerned, specifically the rights of translation, reprinting, reuse of illustrations, recitation, broadcasting, reproduction on microfilms or in any other physical way, and transmission or information storage and retrieval, electronic adaptation, computer software, or by similar or dissimilar methodology now known or hereafter developed.
The use of general descriptive names, registered names, trademarks, service marks, etc. in this publication does not imply, even in the absence of a specific statement, that such names are exempt from the relevant protective laws and regulations and therefore free for general use.
The publisher, the authors and the editors are safe to assume that the advice and information in this book are believed to be true and accurate at the date of publication. Neither the publisher nor the authors or the editors give a warranty, express or implied, with respect to the material contained herein or for any errors or omissions that may have been made. The publisher remains neutral with regard to jurisdictional claims in published maps and institutional affiliations.

Cover illustration: shansekala/gettyimages

Printed on acid-free paper

This Palgrave Macmillan imprint is published by Springer Nature
The registered company is Macmillan Publishers Ltd.
The registered company address is: The Campus, 4 Crinan Street, London, N1 9XW, United Kingdom

'Education either functions as an instrument which is used to facilitate integration of the younger generation into the logic of the present system and bring about conformity or it becomes the practice of freedom, the means by which men and women deal critically and creatively with reality and discover how to participate in the transformation of their world'. (Paulo Freire, 1972: Pedagogy of the Oppressed)

This book is written in the belief that caring nurses are brought into being, not in the form of personality traits, judged through checklists at admission interview, but rather through a form of nursing education that is capable of nurturing students from those same communities which, as qualified nurses, those students will go on to serve. As such, nurses deserve an education as much as any university student and not merely to be professionally trained. It follows that notions of elite nursing or elite nurses are not ones I can condone. Therefore, this book is dedicated not to some nurses but to all nurses, all nurse educators and all nursing students.

Acknowledgements

The idea of exploring and developing ideas around pedagogy in nursing would not have happened without the many educators, students, teachers and practising nurses and midwives who have shaped my thoughts, feelings and understanding of education over a long career. In recent years though, I have had time, previously taken up by teaching and by curriculum development, to reflect on my own educational practices and those of my colleagues, being in the fortunate position to concentrate on researching and thinking about learning and teaching in nursing. For this opportunity I thank all my colleagues at Middlesex University. Whether they are aware of it or not, nevertheless I am eternally grateful.

While I recognise my limitations as a writer and researcher, having come late to the party so to speak, I am grateful to my husband Simon Dyson for his ability to see around my oft less than fully formed ideas, and for offering suggestions as to how to develop the arguments further and to articulate what I believe is an essential consideration for nurse education, namely, the potential for transformative pedagogy to shape the nursing curriculum. This is of great importance for me in that as a doctor of education, I consider education to be my practice, but as a nurse and midwife, it is also important that I should articulate a view of nurse education as praxis.

Special thanks will always go to Emma von Pahlen and Matthew McCartney. I could not have written this book without their continued love and support and I thank them both.

Thank you also to Rehana and Ingrid Dyson. The special nature of the stepmother/stepdaughter relationship is known only to those who have traversed it and come out the other side the better for it. I would not have wanted it any other way and could not now imagine my life without them in it.

Lastly, special thanks to Nina whose very presence in my life has led to my own shift in meaning perspective. Having a grandchild is a life-changing event and has been for me a game changer.

Contents

1	Introduction	1
2	Nursing, Nurse Education and the National Health Service: A Tripartite Relationship	21
3	Global Health and Global Nurse Education	53
4	Pedagogy in Nurse Education	69
5	Transforming Nurse Education	97
6	Co-creation in Nurse Education	121
7	Preparing Nurses for Contemporary Nursing Practice	139
	References	173
	Index	187

List of Figures

Fig. 7.1	Product/Process Curriculum Models	162
Fig. 7.2	Spiral Curriculum Model	163
Fig. 7.3	Combined Process/Spiral Curriculum Model	164
Fig. 7.4	Volunteering as Pedagogy in a Combined Process/Spiral Curriculum Model	165

List of Tables

Table 7.1	Facilitated reflection on a volunteering activity	158
Table 7.2	Levels of reflection on a volunteering activity	160

1

Introduction

Most people reading this book will know only too well of the scandal surrounding Mid Staffordshire NHS Foundation Trust, whereby poor care between 2005 and 2009 reportedly contributed to the avoidable deaths of many patients. The public inquiry which followed cost the taxpayer £13 million, interviewed more than 160 witnesses, sifted through one million pages of evidence and resulted in 290 recommendations contained within a four-volume report that stretched over 1800 pages (Kapur, 2014). Failings were identified at every level including individuals, management, regulators of nursing, the nursing profession and nurse education (Francis, 2013). The inquiry drew on the oral accounts and written witness statements of almost 300 patients and families, before concluding that nurses at the hospital lacked the skills to care and the inherent qualities to do so with compassion. While any criticism of the profession is difficult to accept, failings in compassionate care are particularly concerning, given the defining characteristics of nursing include "to respect the dignity, autonomy and uniqueness of human beings" (RCN, 2003, p. 3). There is no doubt that emphasis needs to be placed on care and compassion in nursing, for these are fundamental values underpinning nursing. In this respect, the public have a right to expect, when admitted to hospital or when receiving nursing care in the community, that they will be treated with the dignity and respect they deserve. With that said, there needs also to be an acknowledgement of the contextual factors impacting nursing work, for example perceived autonomy or lack thereof, involvement in decision-making, workload issues, and associated stress and burnout (Wallin, Ewald, Wikblad, Scott-Finley, & Arnetz, 2006). Without such acknowledgement, it is difficult for nurse education to conceptualise nursing in such a way as to ameliorate the factors impacting the ability of nurses to provide high-quality care, and to do so with compassion.

Nurse education needs to play its part in preparing nurses who are able to respond appropriately when nursing values are called into question. Critical thinking skills and critically reflective practice are essential tools for contemporary nursing practice and should therefore be an integral component of the nursing curriculum. This requires nurse educators to have knowledge of theories and practice in curriculum development in order to ensure nursing programmes prepare nurses who demonstrate competency in practice, alongside caring and compassionate behaviours and attitudes.

The premise on which this book rests is for a mindful consideration of pedagogy in nursing to sit alongside the measures taken by the government, by the Nursing and Midwifery Council (NMC) and by the Council of Deans of Health (CoDH) to address the issue of quality of care in nursing. This introduction begins by examining the response to the Francis Inquiry from the National Health Service (NHS), the Royal College of Nursing (RCN), the CoDH and the NMC, within the context of their impact on discourse around care, compassion, values based recruitment (VBR) and apprenticeships in nursing. The chapter introduces the notion of transformative pedagogy in nurse education as a leitmotif throughout the book.

The National Health Service

The response of the NHS to the Francis Report was immediate, with most healthcare organisations accepting the recommendations and instigating changes in the short, medium and long term. The Nuffield Trust, in research carried out within a year of the report's publication, found the

Francis Report has been taken very seriously by those working in NHS acute trusts. Furthermore, "the welfare of patients and high quality care was uppermost in their minds" (Nuffield Trust, 2014, p. 37). The Nuffield Trust, while recognising the limitations of the research, which provided a glimpse of activity and views of one-third of hospital trusts, nevertheless concluded that it remains to be seen whether the Francis Report will result in measurably improved care for patients and how extensive this will be across hospital trusts more generally. Critical to this is the fundamental tension between commitments to care quality, safe staffing and zero harm, on the one hand, and the relentless financial constraints facing the NHS for the foreseeable future, on the other (Nuffield Trust, 2014, p. 44).

The Royal College of Nursing

The RCN is the world's largest nursing union and professional body, representing more than 435,000 nurses, student nurses, midwives and healthcare assistants in the UK and internationally. Governed by an elected council of 31 members, who delegate the running and management of the organisation to a Chief Executive and General Secretary, the RCN is a Royal Charter body registered with the Privy Council. Along with normal trade union activities, for example negotiating pay terms and conditions for NHS staff and staff working within independent sector organisations, the RCN, through its lobby activities, influences governments and other bodies across the UK to develop, influence and implement policy to improve the quality of patient care (RCN, 2016). With respect to the Francis Report's recommendations concerning nurse education, in particular the call for prospective nursing students to spend up to three months working on direct patient care under the supervision of a qualified nurse, the RCN responded by stating:

> we firmly believe that the 2300 hours that student nurses currently spend on clinical placements is sufficient preparation for the world of practice and patient care. Furthermore, there is no evidence that newly qualified nurses are exhibiting any behaviours that should give rise to the kinds of concerns that would warrant such a radical change to the current system. (RCN, 2013a, p. 6)

The RCN, in this respect, shared the view of the Willis Commission on the future of nurse education, who saw no major shortcomings in the way future nurses are trained (Willis, 2012). Irrespective of the RCN's confidence in the current system, stakeholders in nurse education have a duty to consider the efficacy of the current system in preparing nurses for the emotional burden of their work (Proctor, Wallbank, & Dhaliwal, 2013).

The Council of Deans of Health

The CoDH represents the UK's university faculties engaged in education and research for nurses, midwives and allied health professionals. Considered to be the voice of the professions, the CoDH operates across the UK at the heart of policy and political debate (www.councilofdeans. org.uk). In a discussion paper on educating the future nurse, the CoDH suggests that developing clear competencies for the newly graduated nurse is a significant opportunity to articulate the value and contribution of the profession. However, at the same time, the CoDH highlights the limitations of competency-based models and the risk of creating a formulaic, box-ticking educational culture, which stifles innovation and creativity (CoDH, 2016).

The Nursing and Midwifery Council

The NMC is the regulator of nurses, midwives and health visitors in the UK, whose primary purpose is to protect the public by setting standards of education, training, conduct and performance. The NMC holds the register for all nurses who have qualified and meet the standards. In addition, the NMC is responsible for fair and effective fitness to practice processes to investigate and deal with nurses and midwives who fall short of the standards. With respect to nurse education, the NMC responded to the first Francis Independent Inquiry in 2010 by publishing new standards for preregistration nurse education, which placed significant emphasis on care and compassion for patients. The NMC's response to the Francis Report of 2013 concentrated on issues concerning healthcare assistants and support workers, on complaints, on professional regulation and on safety (NMC, 2013).

Care and Compassion in Nursing

Since the Francis Report 'care and compassion' has become a trope, a figure of speech, used in this instance to support the speakers (undeclared) neoliberal agenda. In other words, a call to reform both the NHS and nurse education, by claiming neither is fit for the purpose in the twenty-first century. The problem with putting the words together compels the reader to attend to both concepts as psychological traits or behavioural tendencies held (or not held) by individuals: a nurse is either a caring and compassionate individual, or they are not, as the case might be. This enables the 'problem' to lie within the individual and not with organisational factors, which ultimately determine how health services are organised, managed and delivered. On the other hand, if care is viewed as physical labour, emotional labour and organisation then 'care' is more than attitude. Nurses may or may not have control over the flow, pace and indeed goals of the work they undertake. Context may determine if emotional labour compromises the capacity of nurses to undertake care in a compassionate manner. The organisation necessary for care determines whether the nurse has the positive freedom to care, whether they have the resources and infrastructure to undertake care work (James, 1992).

The current trend to engage in dialogue intrinsically coupling care with compassion has resulted in a blame culture, whereby nurse practitioners point the figure at nurse education, and nurse educators reciprocate by pointing to poor nursing practice (Bewley, 2016). Apportioning blame is a falsely reassuring response to quality issues (Baker, 2015). Blame is a comforting but counterproductive reaction when attached to quality failures. Blaming nurse education and nursing practice for quality failures supports prescriptive approaches to nurse education, evidenced by redevelopment of standards for preregistration nurse education (NMC, 2010), revalidation for qualified practitioners (NMC, 2016a) and a focus on VBR (HEE, 2016).

Compassion in nursing practice is a complex phenomenon to describe, in that it is entirely subjective with everyone, be it patients, nurses and politicians having a personal, subjective view of what constitutes compassionate nursing practice. This raises obvious difficulties for nurse education in that views as to what is and is not compassionate practice will drive particular agendas and polices. For example, if compassionate practice rests on the ability of nurses to demonstrate technologically advanced practice then nurse education needs to ensure these skills are embedded within nursing programmes. However, if compassionate practice rests on the ability of nurses to demonstrate highly developed communication skills, then this also needs to be evident within the nursing curriculum. Of course, these are of equal importance within the nursing curriculum, alongside other skills such as an understanding of innovation and research. However, contextual issues often impact the ability for compassionate practice to become a transferable skill for nurses, for example lack of time, lack of resources, increased levels of stress and burnout. In times such as these, instrumental caring, which includes the required skills and knowledge, and expressive caring involving the emotional aspects of the relationship may be compromised, which might explain but not justify the events at Mid Staffordshire NHS Foundation Trust.

It may be argued that nurse educators have a responsibility to identify applicants to nursing programmes who can demonstrate the characteristics of compassion. However, this is extremely difficult to do given the subjective nature of compassion and the fact that these characteristics are not in themselves clear (Proctor et al., 2013). How a student might go about proving herself/himself to be a compassionate individual is at least as difficult as a nurse educator's task in reviewing the evidence. Even if it were possible to make a reasonable attempt to assess the presence or not, as the case might be, of characteristics of compassion within a potential nursing student, whether it is acceptable to reject a potential student on this basis is questionable. Admission to nursing programmes does not require students to demonstrate advance knowledge of technologies in nursing, or anatomy and physiology, rather ensuring this is covered in the curriculum. It is reasonable therefore to suggest nursing programmes take the same approach to learning and teaching about compassion. The problem, however, lies in how this is taught and how the efficacy of such teaching is evaluated upon completion of the programme. It is for these reasons, that other approaches to the identification of a predisposition towards compassion have been promulgated, for example VBR.

Values Based Recruitment in Nursing

VBR is an approach which attracts and selects students on the basis that their individual values and behaviours align with the values of the NHS constitution. The NHS constitution establishes the principles and values of the NHS in England, and sets out rights to which patients, public and staff are entitled. Health Education England (HEE), which works across England to deliver high-quality education and training, has a statutory duty to promote the NHS constitution. HEE's work on VBR is to promote and support the embedding of the values of the NHS Constitution in healthcare, education and training (HEE, 2016).

A major problem with the notion of VBR in nursing and midwifery is that this individualises an issue that is more adequately conceptualised as about social relations. Chattoo and Ahmad (2008) demonstrate that care is an emergent property of social relationships, therefore the potential for caring cannot be reduced to alleged qualities residing inside the person. In addition, values, and how these are enacted, are likely to vary according to class, gender and ethnicity (Skeggs, 2014). Thus, the focus on VBR not only ignores the social relations at play in contemporary nursing practice, but also perpetuates the idea that nurses are in control of the context in which they practice. The focus on the values agenda across the NHS ignores organisational factors which impact quality of care. VBR is a response to concerns raised by the Francis Inquiry that nurses lack the behaviours consistent with caring and compassionate practice. However, VBR is by its very nature, a behaviourist framework. The locus of control over events and outcomes, including how care is delivered and in what manner is seen to reside internally with the individual nurse, as opposed to externally whereby outside forces impact events and their outcomes, which are in effect outside the control of the individual nurse.

Contextual Issues in Nurse Education

Traditional models of nurse education were based on an apprenticeship model, which saw nurses learning by doing: on the job, under the control of skilled practitioners (Aldrich, 2006). Nursing students, within an apprenticeship framework were inducted into a community of nursing practice, with learning taking place in a 'safe environment', guided by 'expert practitioners'. While the apprenticeship model has long declined in nursing, with hospital-based training replaced by 'academy-based' education, nevertheless nurse education is redolent of apprenticeship, for example reliance on mentorship by registered practitioners, and provision of a safe learning environment (all clinical placements used in undergraduate nursing programmes are subject to audit for suitability by participating; Approved Education Institutions, QAA, 2015). The current context of healthcare clearly impacts the concept of safe environment and expert practitioner as evidenced by the Francis Inquiry and other similar reports, which recognise the relationship between quality of care and availability of qualified nurses (Ball, Murrells, Rafferty, Morrow, & Griffiths, 2013). However, it is within this context that the current government is considering introducing apprenticeships in nursing, midwifery and the allied professions.

Nationally, the apprenticeship agenda is rapidly gaining pace. The government is committed to achieving three million apprenticeships by 2020 as part of its productivity agenda. With the introduction of the employees' apprenticeship levy due to start in April 2017 all employers with a UK pay bill of over £3 million, including higher education institutions (public and private), will be required to pay 0.5% of the pay bill into a levy, which is then ring fenced via an electronic voucher system to purchase apprenticeship training (BPP, 2016). While apprenticeships in the wider economy have, up to this point, been below degree level, the emphasis is now on the development of degree level apprenticeships, which by definition will include undergraduate degrees in nursing and midwifery.

The government's ambitions around nursing apprenticeships raise a number of concerns for nursing and midwifery, not least the requirement for end-point assessment (EPA). EPA is a new way of assuring quality in the apprenticeship system, replacing the existing model of continuous assessment resulting in qualifications. Clearly EPA has major implications for degrees in nursing and midwifery, which rely almost entirely on continuous assessment in line with NMC standards. Degree level apprenticeships which will result in a degree awarded by a university (which is subject to QA) and, in the case of nursing, tied to rigorous NMC standards could potentially be at odds with EPA carried out by employers (CoDH, 2016).

EPA of nursing apprenticeship programmes, should it be carried out by the NHS, will need to take account of the conditions of the workplace, whereby skilled staff are in short supply, and where heavy reliance on agency and international nurses often results in priority given to upskilling the registered workforce (Allan & Larson, 2003). Notwithstanding the government's plans around apprenticeships nurses have a right to expect nurse education should equip them with knowledge and skills to enable them to recognise, examine and address the issues in the contemporary nursing workplace. In view of this nurse educators have a responsibility to carefully determine pedagogy and to design nursing curricula to enable students to not only practice competently, but know the important distinction between what is 'good enough' and what should not be tolerated. Critical pedagogy for nurse education is the means by which nurses are educated to not only know this difference, but also have the skills to act when care is unacceptable and be assured that concerns about care, raised in good faith, will be robustly addressed.

Pedagogy in Nurse Education

Pedagogy in nurse education is concerned with what nurses need to know in order to understand nursing as a social enterprise, as a political activity and as a technically demanding profession in an age where patients, families and carers have access to medical- and health-related information on a global scale. The goal of nurse education is thus to prepare nurses to meet the challenges of contemporary nursing practice. However, despite this rhetoric, pedagogy in nurse education has not kept pace with societal, organisational and technological change. Instead nurse education displays elements of apprenticeship style training reminiscent of nurse training prior to the reforms of the early 1990s, commonly termed 'Project 2000' whereby the academic level of training was established at a minimum of a higher education diploma (Eaton, 2012). The NMC, in its response to the initial Francis Inquiry's concerns around nurses' apparent lack of skills and behaviours for compassionate care, has revisited standards for initial nurse education while at the same time remaining committed to an outcomes driven competency-based framework. This, together with the government's focus on behaviourist approaches to nursing recruitment, has resulted in a restricted, as opposed to elaborated language or code (Bernstein, 1971) on which to base nursing pedagogy. The language concerning nurse education, for example standards, competencies and VBR, reflects the assumptions of the protagonists, namely government and the NMC. As a result, nurse educators have little opportunity to explore the potential for critical pedagogies to transform nurse education. This book argues that in times of uncertainty around healthcare policy and subsequent healthcare provision nurse educators are constrained by conventional approaches to curriculum design, which no longer serve nurse education well.

This Book

The book will be of interest to nurse educators, working within higher education, who are interested to develop the nursing curriculum in ways which will enable nurses to meet the challenges of twenty-first-century healthcare, but where patients, client and their families deserve the highest standards of care. A romanticised view of nursing will not suffice in the current climate. Nurses need to be educated to recognise what constitutes acceptable care and what should not be tolerated, and to know the difference. This is a key concept within the book and is addressed through a detailed and critical exploration of innovative nursing pedagogies.

The book will also be of interest to practitioners, educators and student nurses interested to understand why the theory–practice gap in nursing persists, despite attempts over time to reform nurse education. The book takes a unique approach in detailing the current context for healthcare in the UK, before drawing together accounts of healthcare systems around the world, with particular attention to how nurse education is organised to meet local need.

Throughout the book, the notion of transformative pedagogy as antidote to the criticisms levelled at nursing and nurse education is offered as leitmotif. The book does not suggest these criticisms are misplaced and as such the findings and subsequent recommendations of the Francis Inquiry are accepted here, in the same way as others have done so. The book does however concern itself with ways in which a mindful consideration of alternative, namely, transformative pedagogy have potential to address the concern that nurse education is no longer able to guarantee the preparation of nurses who have the necessary knowledge and skills, and behaviours consistent with caring and compassionate practice. To this end, the book offers a critical appraisal of those transformative pedagogies, considered to positively impact the capacity for nurse education to achieve its stated aims and intentions, in order that nurse educators might consider these when planning or redeveloping the nursing curriculum.

The book makes note of the fact that nurse educators, often drawn from clinical practice in recognition of their clinical expertise and its importance to the nursing curriculum, may have limited knowledge of and/or insight into curriculum development and its attendant theories and practices. The book therefore offers guidance on how these theories and practices underpin curriculum development in terms of conceptualisation of nursing and nurse education in the curriculum and how this informs subsequent selection of a curriculum model. Product and process curriculum models are described, along with their attendant properties, before considering how each model might be used in nursing. Nursing as a body of knowledge, as product, as process and as praxis are discussed, before considering the context in which the nursing curriculum is delivered. The book then returns to its central theme of transformative pedagogies by looking in particular at volunteering. When organised within the curriculum, volunteering as pedagogy facilitates critically reflective learning and teaching strategies (narrative, dialogic and case stories), which can lead students to become critically reflective practitioners; hence the curriculum embodies the notion of theory in action, in other words praxis.

Finally, the book revisits the notion of co-creation, offering ideas as to how co-creation might be conceptualised within the nursing curriculum. A co-created model is thus described whereby learners are considered as assets, as agents of change and as active participants in the learning process. To this end a spiral design is proposed, whereby nursing content and concepts are revisited throughout the nursing programme, and where a constructivist approach allows learners to construct hypotheses about nursing in the safe environment of the classroom, wherever that classroom might be located. Volunteering as a structured opportunity within the curriculum is offered as explanation for how the model might work in practice, while at the same time recognising the complexities involved in offering volunteering opportunities to nursing students. The absence of the resources required if volunteering as pedagogy is to become integral to curriculum design does not preclude the use of the model described in this book. Conventional practice components of pre-registration nursing programmes would fit equally well with the concepts underlying the co-created curriculum model. A detailed description of each chapter is offered below:

Chapter 2 provides the basis for a detailed discussion of pedagogy in nurse education in the UK. Factors impacting the design and delivery of nursing programmes are examined, including key relationships between the NMC and the Approved Education Institution. The NMC and nurse education are argued to make for an uneasy alliance, whereby regulation stifles creative pedagogical solutions to the issues facing nurse education in the current climate of political and organisational uncertainty for healthcare services in the UK.

The implied criticism of nurse education in the wake of the Francis Inquiry is argued to have revived debate as to where and how nurses are educated. The discourse around the educational context in which nursing students are taught is framed within a wider debate around care and compassion in nursing, which pays little attention to the contextual factors impacting nursing work. In educational terms the ramifications of this discourse are far reaching, in that nursing as an academic discipline has been traditionally subordinated to medicine. Location of nursing within higher education went some way towards redressing the balance; therefore, relocation of nursing into the practice setting is seen as a retrograde step.

The current context of healthcare services is suggested to have severely impacted the capacity for nurses to think creatively, and to arrive at solutions to problems of finite resources, staff shortages and rising public expectation in terms of diagnosis, treatment, acute and long-term care. The chapter suggests the need for innovative and transformative pedagogies for nurse education, as a considered response to reported failure of nurses to provide care with compassion. The chapter begins a pressing dialogue concerning innovative and transformative pedagogy for nurse education, which is vital in the wake of the public inquiry into failings in care at Mid Staffordshire NHS Foundation Trust. The current context of healthcare services is argued to severely impact the capacity for nurses to think creatively, and to arrive at solutions to problems of finite resources, staff shortages and rising public expectation in terms of diagnosis, treatment, acute and long-term care. The chapter introduces the concept of co-production in healthcare as *leitmotif* in this book. Parallels are drawn between the principles of co-production and co-creation.

Chapter 3 discusses global health services and ways in which nurse education has developed to meet local needs. The way in which healthcare is organised across the globe is argued to depend on the wealth of the country under consideration. All industrialised nations, with the exception of the USA, implement some form of universal healthcare, with the main ways including government run (tax funded) systems, for example the NHS; privately run but government pays the lions share, for example Canada and France; and private insurance arrangements such as exists in Switzerland. The USA does not provide universal healthcare for all citizens, but has programmes for the elderly, military service families, the disabled, children and some poor through Medicare and Medicaid, with the result that around 45 million people in the USA are either uninsured or underinsured. In developing countries, that is those considered not wealthy, while some strive to provide universal healthcare, most struggle to do so due to lack of resources, inappropriate use of resources or misappropriation of resources to fund war and conflict. Increasing longevity coupled with exponential increases in long-term, complex health conditions, is argued as a global phenomenon, causing governments worldwide to rethink how healthcare is conceptualised and subsequently funded.

The chapter makes connections between demographic changes, population growth, global health needs and the impact of migration of the nursing workforce, drawing on recent evidence around the experience of the overseas nursing workforce in the UK, and the implications for practice and education. Disparity between nations with respect to provision of healthcare services is replicated in approaches to nurse education, with the length of nursing programmes seen to vary from two to five years, with some differences noted in arrangements for midwifery education. Actions taken by the World Health Organisation (WHO) to address disparities between healthcare programmes are described, namely efforts to standardise nursing and midwifery education across member countries and the impact of this on migration of the healthcare workforce.

Chapter 4 considers pedagogy in nurse education. The chapter begins with an overview of historical developments in nurse education. The transference of nurse education into higher education is argued to have failed in its aspirations to intellectualise nurse education due to constraints around regulation and curriculum design. Critical pedagogy is suggested as an antidote to conventional approaches to learning and teaching nursing. The work of Paolo Freire and Henry Giroux is considered of particular relevance for nurse education, as both offer insight into ways of thinking about present-day, modern nursing, which takes account of the social, political and technological context of healthcare. The chapter argues for 'pedagogically appropriate' nurse education, as a suitable response to the concerns and criticisms of both the nursing workforce and the nurse education. Jack Mezirow's work on adult learning provides a critical lens through which to view the role of the nursing curriculum in the development of sustainable positive nursing practice. Critical thinking is considered fundamental to contemporary nursing work and key to development of knowledgeable, competent, caring and compassionate practice. The chapter considers ways in which key components of critical thinking: critical reading, critical writing, critical listening and critical speaking can be incorporated into the nursing curriculum.

Chapter 5 builds on the principles of co-production discussed in Chap. 2 by considering ways in which transformative pedagogies can be incorporated into contemporary nursing curricula through co-productive approaches to education. Transformative pedagogy is argued to empower students through appropriate teaching methods to effect change and to enable them to make sense of contemporary nursing practice.

The chapter begins by suggesting that the 'hidden curriculum' effectively contributes to a persistent theory–practice gap, whereby students' report what is taught in theory is often not enacted in practice. Students are often taught an idealised version of nursing, which cannot be accommodated in the real-life social settings in which nursing work occurs. The chapter argues for a nursing curriculum, which draws on different types of nursing knowledge, to ensure aspects of professionalism, traditionally hidden within the curriculum, are made explicit and subject to critical examination.

The chapter advances the argument that nurse education in attempting to address inherent criticisms of the nursing profession has not focused attention on critical pedagogies, nor how these impact the potential for the nursing curriculum to equip nurses with critical awareness, socially conscious practice, and cognitive and affective understanding of the social, political and technological context of healthcare practice. This chapter moves beyond the rhetoric in suggesting nurse educators have a responsibility to ensure nursing programmes are designed and delivered in ways, which maximise the potential for nursing students to develop the attributes necessary for present-day, modern nursing. Consideration is given to the role of the hidden curriculum, whereby nursing students are often left to internalise professional values consistent with nursing practice, as opposed to explicit consideration within the curriculum, so much so that the theory–practice gap persists in nursing and is of perennial concern for nursing students. The chapter considers the need for the nursing curriculum to draw on different types of nursing knowledge, in order to illuminate aspects of nursing traditionally hidden from students, but which are key for helping students to bridge the theory–practice gap, in other words to make sense of contemporary nursing practice, for example a constructivist approach, whereby students are encouraged to constantly assess how each learning activity is assisting their understanding. The chapter considers the practical application of a spiral curriculum, as a means for combining constructivism with critical pedagogy.

The final section in this chapter expands on the principles of co-production first discussed in Chap. 2, paying attention to its application to nurse education. Co-creation and co-design are argued as more appropriate concepts when thinking about developing the nursing curriculum, in that their use ensures the full range of activities is encompassed, as opposed to a focus on the end point or outcome. This chapter builds on the principles of co-production discussed in an earlier chapter by considering ways in which transformative pedagogy can be incorporated into contemporary nursing curricula through co-creative approaches to education.

Chapter 6 develops the concept of co-creation within nurse education. The discussion positions students as a key resource within nurse education, for reasons that the statutory body for the regulation of nurse education in the UK, the NMC requires students to spend 50% of their learning in the practice setting. This requirement invariably means nursing students accrue practice experience, which is often both more contextual and more current than that of the nurse educators who are teaching them. Despite this, nursing students are rarely, if ever, consulted about their educational experiences with a view to informing the nursing curriculum, although they will be assessed in practice on the achievement of clinical competency. While many nurse educators engage in co-creation this is usually confined to activities at the level of the classroom, and as such is limited to learning and teaching methods, with the result that co-creation does not permeate curriculum development in any meaningful sense. The chapter suggests this represents a lost opportunity to engage students in the designing of teaching approaches, courses and content, in other words co-creation of the curriculum, in ways which would harness the potential for students to move from passivity to agency, a shift which is crucial in the current context of the NHS.

The chapter considers how the notion of the co-created curriculum challenges conventional conceptions of learners as subordinate to the expert tutor in engaging with what is taught and how it is taught. The chapter, notwithstanding the challenges in enacting co-creation principles in education, regards students as agents in the process of transformative learning, whereby the aim is to strive for radical collegiality in relation to course content and approaches to learning and teaching. The chapter suggests co-creation in the nursing curriculum has potential to assist students with the transition from enacting what is required of them in order to complete the study programme (the nursing degree), to consciously analyse what constitutes and enhances that learning, that is what the learner knows, to who the learner is.

Chapter 7 considers what nurse educators can do to design and deliver a nursing curriculum fit for the purpose of preparing nurses for the challenge of contemporary nursing practice. The challenges facing nurse educators are argued as multifactorial and complex, thus strengthening the case for consideration of alternative pedagogies for nursing. The chapter acknowledges recent efforts by the NMC to strengthen public confidence in the profession, through an enhanced system of appraisal, whereby the onus is placed on nurses and midwives to demonstrate continued ability to practise safely and effectively. The chapter considers the likelihood of success of these measures in light of criticism of the underlying principles and practices pertaining to appraisal. The chapter recognises, notwithstanding the validity of concerns raised over the process of revalidation, the NMC is clearly concerned to protect patient safety and to support a culture of professionalism, thus arguing for nurse education to work alongside the NMC to design nursing programmes, which can guarantee public trust and confidence in the graduate nurse.

The chapter begins by considering the complex contextual issues facing health and social care, and the challenges posed therein for curriculum development in a climate of uncertainty. The argument is made for nurse educators to demonstrate familiarity with theories and practices underpinning curriculum development as pre-requisite for the role. To this end, the chapter offers a detailed discussion of approaches to conceptualising the nursing curriculum, including curriculum as product, as process and as praxis. This section concludes with a discussion of the nursing curriculum in context, which recognises the multifactorial context for nurse education. Practical consideration is given to what nurse educators can do to design and deliver a nursing curriculum fit for the purpose of preparing nurses for contemporary nursing practice. To this end, a model for contemporary nurse education is described, which draws together the key arguments in this book, that is critical pedagogy as a transformative agent, and structured opportunities for volunteering as a means of engaging the nursing curriculum in the co-creation imperative.

References

Aldrich, R. (2006). *Lessons from history of education*. London: Routledge.

Allan, H. T., & Larsen, J. A. (2003). *"We need respect": Experiences of internationally recruited nurses in the UK*. London: RCN.

Baker, E. (2015). Transparency will only change culture if we eradicate blame as a response. Retrieved December 9, 2016, from http://www.cqc.org.uk/content/transparency-will-only-change-culture-if-we-eradicate-blame-response

Ball, J. E., Murrells, T., Rafferty, A., Morrow, E., & Griffiths, P. (2013, July 29). Care left undone during nursing shifts: Associations with workload and perceived quality of care. *BMJ Quality and Safety*, Online First. Retrieved November 30, 2016, from http://qualitysafety.bmj.com/

Bernstein, B. (1971). *Class, codes and control* (Vol. 1). London: Kegan Paul.

Bewley, A. (2016). Is education to blame for safeguarding failures. *Nursing Standard, 30*(19), 32–33.

BPP. (2016). The apprenticeship levy – Opportunities for your business. Retrieved December 2, 2016, from www.bpp.com

Chattoo, S., & Ahmad, W. I. U. (2008). The moral economy of selfhood and caring: Negotiating boundaries of personal care as embodied moral practice. *Sociology of Health & Illness, 30*(4), 550–564.

Council of Deans of Health. (2016). Educating the future nurse – A paper for discussion. Retrieved November 9, 2016, from www.councilofdeans.org.uk

Eaton, A. (2012). Pre-registration nurse education: A brief history. Retrieved December 8, 2016, from www.williscommission.org.uk

Francis, R. (2013). *Report of the Mid Staffordshire NHS Foundation Trust public inquiry*. London: The Stationery Office.

HEE. (2016). Values based recruitment framework. Health Education England. Retrieved December 9, 2016, from https://www.hee.nhs.uk/…/values-based-recruitment

James, N. (1992). Care = organisation + physical labour + emotional labour. *Sociology of Health & Illness, 14*, 488–509.

Kapur, N. (2014). Mid Staffordshire Hospital report: What does psychology have to offer. *The Psychologist, 27*, 16–20.

NMC. (2010). *Standards for pre-registration nurse education*. London: NMC.

NMC. (2013). NMC response to the Francis report. The response of the Nursing and Midwifery Council to the Mid Staffordshire NHS Foundation Trust Public Inquiry report. 18 July 2016. Retrieved December 7, 2016, from http://www.nmc.org.uk/globalassets/sitedocuments/francis-report/nmc-response

References

NMC. (2016a). *Revalidation*. Retrieved December 9, 2016, from http://revalidation.nmc.org.uk/

Proctor, S., Wallbank, S., & Dhaliwal, J. S. (2013). What compassionate care means. Retrieved December 3, 2016, from www.hsj.co.uk/comment/what-compassionate-care-means/5055438.artile

Quality Assurance Agency (QAA). (2015). The quality code. Retrieved from www.qaa.ac.uk

RCN. (2003, republished 2014). *Defining nursing*. London: RCN. Online. Retrieved December 3, 2016, from www.rcn.org.uk

RCN. (2013). *Mid Staffordshire NHS Foundation Trust. Response of the Royal College of Nursing*. London: RCN. www.rcn.org.uk

RCN. (2016). *What the RCN does*. London: RCN. Retrieved December 7, 2016, from http://www.rcn.org.uk/about-us/what-the-rcn-does

Skeggs, B. (2014). Values beyond value? Is anything beyond the logic of capital? *British Journal of Sociology, 65*(1), 1–20.

The Nuffield Trust. (2014). The Francis report: One year on. Retrieved December 7, 2016, from www.nuffiledtrust.org.uk

Wallin, R., Ewald, U., Wikblad, K., Scott-Finley, S., & Arnetz, B. (2006). Understandings work contextual factors: A short-cut to evidence-based practice? *Evidence-Based Nursing, 3*(4), 153–164.

Willis Commission. (2012). *Quality with compassion: The future of nurse education*. Report of the Willis Commission, London: RCN. Retrieved from www.williscommission.org.uk

2

Nursing, Nurse Education and the National Health Service: A Tripartite Relationship

Introduction

Concerns around quality of care in nursing have opened nurse education up to public scrutiny. Deficiencies in training and inadequate experience throughout the nursing programme are seen as reasons for nurse *education*, currently located within higher education, to be replaced with nurse *training*, located within practice settings, namely the National Health Service (NHS). This argument is essentially captured in the notion that nurses are too posh to wash and too clever to care (Scott, 2004). The environment in which nurses' work to a large extent determines the quality and safety of the care patients receive. Consequently, when care falls short of standards nurses' shoulder much of the responsibility, irrespective of the contextual factors impacting nursing work, for example resource allocation, workfoce issues or lack of appropriate polices (Hughes, 2008). Uncertainty around healthcare policy impacts the capacity for nurse education to respond to social, economic and political uncertainty, through recourse to innovative and creative pedagogies for nursing, in part due to requirements for undergraduate programmes to comply with rigorous Nursing and Midwifery Council (NMC) standards for undergraduate nursing programmes. As such, the potential for critical pedagogies to transform nurse education is severely limited (Ironside, 2001). A prescriptive approach, whereby all learners undertake the same programme, with limited attention paid to prior experiential learning (certificated or non-certificated), impacts possibilities for undergraduate nursing programmes to address concerns around quality of nursing care through educational strategies and solutions, in particular through transformative critical pedagogies for nursing. Nurse educators have a responsibility and an opportunity, through careful design and delivery of nursing curricula to prepare nurses to understand complex care processes, complex healthcare technologies, complex patient needs and responses to therapeutic interventions, and complex organisations. The book is therefore particularly concerned with how nurse educators, through mindful consideration of pedagogy, including theory and practice in curriculum development can prepare nursing students for the increasingly complex and challenging situations, which characterise contemporary healthcare environments.

The chapter begins with a consideration of the relationship between the NMC and nurse education, and the subsequent impact of this relationship on nursing pedagogy. The NMC and nurse education are argued to make for an uneasy alliance, whereby regulation stifles creative pedagogical solutions to the issues facing nurse education in the current climate of political and organisational uncertainty for healthcare services in the United Kingdom (UK). The implied criticism of nurse education in the wake of the Francis Inquiry into poor care at Mid Staffordshire NHS Foundation Trust has revived debate as to where and how nurses are educated. The discourse around the educational context in which nursing students are taught is framed within a wider debate around care and compassion in nursing, which pays little attention to the contextual factors impacting nursing work. In educational terms the ramifications of this discourse are far reaching, in that nursing as an academic discipline has been traditionally subordinated to medicine. Location of nursing within higher education went some way towards redressing the balance. Relocation of nursing into the practice setting therefore represents a retrograde step.

Nurse Education and the Nursing and Midwifery Council: An Uneasy Alliance

Recent substantive reform to the NHS has seen expanded patient choice, and liberalisation of the hospital sector with publicly owned hospitals (in England) given additional fiscal and managerial autonomy, while at the same time encouraging hospitals to compete within a market with fixed prices (Cooper, Gibbon, Jones, & McGuire, 2011). Throughout this period of reform, the cost of healthcare has continued to escalate within a context of finite resources and budget constraint. As a consequence, questions are continually raised about resource efficiency and mode of service delivery, with subsequent reform leading to periods of further instability. Instability in the NHS directly impacts the nursing workforce. Cost containment contributes to reductions in numbers of commissioned education and training places, reductions in staff numbers, and reduced training budgets for the nursing workforce, the results of which negatively affect nurse education as it struggles to educate the nursing work force within a climate of uncertainty.

The basic principle in educating for uncertainty is to teach students to think, to dissent, to tolerate and to respect other people (Escotet, 2012). However, if student nurses are to learn to solve complex problems within an uncertain healthcare environment then rigid approaches to nursing pedagogy, that is, conventional approaches to learning and teaching will no longer suffice. Conventional pedagogy in nursing centres on acquisition of competencies, with little, if any, attention to the acquisition of critical thinking skills. This conventional approach has fallen short in recent times as the competency of nurses is called into question, alongside concerns around fitness to practice. In 2014/2015, some 5183 referrals were made to the NMC for fitness to practice investigation, an increase of 10.5% on the previous year (figure includes UK and overseas including European Union (EU)). This number represents 0.6% of registrants (NMC, 2015a). While statisticians might argue given the number of nurses registered with the NMC that this figure is to be expected, others, for example service users, might argue within the context of healthcare services no figure is acceptable.

Perhaps a more interesting figure is the 5% (259) of referrals where the type of allegation leading to referral is classed as lack of competency. This figure gives credence to the NMC's focus on standards for competence and standards for education. However, while the NMC suggest programmes should offer a flexible, blended approach to learning, and draw on the full range of modern learning methods and modes of delivery, nevertheless it is the NMC standards, which determine content and other learning opportunities required within a largely competency-based approach to nursing programmes. Programmes leading to the minimum preregistration qualification for entry onto the NMC register (a degree in nursing), need to comply with the standard 50% theory and 50% practice. This requirement leaves little room for innovation as priority is given over to content, achievement of competency, assessment and progression points, mentoring of students, and opportunities to practice. The inevitable result of a standardised approach to the nursing curriculum results in lack of pedagogical innovation and creativity. Traditional pedagogical approaches have become the mainstay for nurse academics charged with responsibility for designing and delivering education programmes which meet the necessary standards required of an NMC Approved Education Institution (AEI).

Regulation of Nurse Education

The Nursing and Midwifery Council (NMC) are the statutory body charged with approving education institutions to deliver nursing and midwifery education in the UK. In its position as regulator the NMC exists to protect the public. It does this by setting education standards, which shape the content and design of programmes, stating the competences of a nurse and midwife, approving education institutions and maintaining a database of approved programmes (courses). The NMC quality assures approved programmes, registers nurses and midwives when they have successfully completed nursing and midwifery courses, and assesses and ensures the quality of practice placements for students (NMC, 2016b).

The NMC point out it is not responsible for educating or selecting students, which is undertaken by the AEI. However, nursing and midwifery programmes have to conform to the standards set by and monitored by the NMC. Similarly, the NMC claim not to set curricula, not to regulate students and not to assess the ability of practice to support students' learning. The NMC, as a regulator of nursing and midwifery education, enacted through the setting of standards which have to be adhered to, means that, in effect, the selection of students onto programmes, their subsequent education, and their fitness to practice throughout their education and upon completion of the programme is all determined by the NMC, albeit devolved to the AEI.

The NMC claims the assessment of the ability of practice settings to support students' learning is the responsibility of the AEI, which is true in principle as AEI's undertake to assess and monitor that practice settings can provide appropriate and timely learning opportunities for students. However, the NMC stipulate that nursing and midwifery programmes must contain 50% of learning in practice. While AEI's by proxy assess practice learning settings, Standard 10 of the NMC Standards for Pre-Registration Education sets out in detail what practice learning opportunities should include, therefore it is the NMC who determine all matters relating to practice learning opportunities and indeed all matters relating to nursing and midwifery education. The only non-contentious statement regarding the role of the NMC in regulating nursing and midwifery education relates to the absence of any role in assessing the quality of care in hospitals or the community, as this is the responsibility of the Care Quality Commission (CQC) in England, Healthcare Improvement Scotland, Healthcare Inspectorate Wales and Northern Ireland's Regulation and Quality Improvement Authority (NMC, 2016b).

The NMC has been subject to intense scrutiny in recent years for its leadership, governance, decision-making and organisation management, culminating in the Council for Healthcare Regulatory Excellence (CHRE) report in 2012. CHRE concluded that the role of the regulator is to set the 'baseline', the standard below which professional practice must not fall and in this, the NMC has not understood its regulatory purpose well, focusing instead on its work on standards and policy. In other words, a focus on standard setting in education culminated in underinvestment in fitness to practise, which is arguably, the rightful role of the regulator (CHRE, 2012). The NMC were also heavily criticised for failings in its handling of cases relating to Mid Staffordshire NHS Foundation Trust. However, more recently the Professional Standards Authority (PSA) has continued to review performance of the NMC, finding improvement in all areas of its functions (PSA, 2014/2015).

In drawing attention to the relationship between the NMC and AEI's, the point is not to criticise the role of the NMC as regulator seeking to protect the public. This regulatory function is both necessary and welcome. Nevertheless, the NMC, in determining both educational standards and regulation, provides for a conflict of interest whereby the primary interest, that is, regulation, impacts on the secondary interest, that is, educational development of nursing curricula, ultimately constraining nurse academics to develop nurse education within a behaviourist, outcome driven and essentially positivist educational framework.

Nursing and Midwifery Council Standards for Preregistration Nursing Programmes

In January 2016, the NMC approved plans to undertake a review of the competencies for new nurses entering the profession to replace the current standards, which were published in 2010 and to which all preregistration nursing programmes adhere. Following an independent evaluation of these standards varying levels of understanding were reported alongside a consensus that the standards were overly complex and too focused on processes rather than outcomes (Macleod Clark, 2016). In light of this, the Council of Deans of Health were asked to advise on the development of the new standards, which the NMC anticipate all institutions will adopt from September 2019, although some institutions will have the option to become early adopters from September 2018. The Council of Deans of Health identify the key skills required of the nursing workforce, namely critical thinking, ability to use advanced technology, to work flexibly and accountably across care settings, to be excellent communicators, and to be able to take the lead in managing complex care packages (CoDH, 2016). Clearly, the future registered nurse must be equipped with the transferable skills that underpin critical thinking, problem solving and decision-making if they are to function at the level required for contemporary nursing practice. However, the manner in which these skills are achieved is as important as achievement of the standards, that is, process is at least as important as outcome. While standards have a necessary place in nurse education, these should not be at the expense of each student's unique learning experience. To ignore the diverse abilities and expectations of nursing students is to ignore the potential for students to engage with the learning process (Wittek and Kvernbekk, 2011). It is only through the educational process as well as achievement of the standards that students come to understand the complexities of healthcare systems and the unique contribution of nursing to decision-making and quality of care. Positionality, that is, the relationship between theory, practice, process and outcome, is an essential element of curriculum design in nurse education (Dyson, Liu, van den Akker, & O'Driscoll, 2017).

Health Services in the UK

There is no such thing as the perfect health system (Britnell, 2015), although governments around the world continue to search for the perfect system within the diverse contexts in which they govern. While a number of different models or approaches to financing healthcare are evident across the globe (taxation, private healthcare insurance and social health insurance) few countries operate any one model in its purest form, with most countries typically adopting an eclectic approach towards payment for healthcare services. The dominant model in any one country is usually a result of historical approaches and ideological beliefs about healthcare funding, mitigated by current political and contextual issues.

In the UK, universal healthcare is funded through a blend of general taxation (76%) and national insurance or payroll tax (18%) and a small number of copayments including charges for prescriptions (Britnell, 2015). However, while the NHS is generally thought of as being free at the point of use, patients in the UK have been required since 1951 to contribute towards the cost of some services, for example prescriptions and dental treatment, although exemptions are in place for people under 16 and over 60, in addition to being free to recipients of some state benefits. As a result of these exemptions, as much as 90% of all prescription items in England have been dispensed free of charge in recent years (Health and Social Care Information Centre, 2016). As an adjunct, the UK population is at liberty to purchase private healthcare insurance or is able to access private insurance through remuneration packages offered by employers, although this is by no means available to all and notwithstanding individual choice, nevertheless raises moral and ethical concerns. Private health insurance, by allowing choice for users is thought to encourage competition and thus drive up standards of care. However, private health insurance discriminates against those on lower incomes, who inversely tend to have a higher need for healthcare. As there is no link between pricing of premiums and personal income, private health insurance invariably costs those on lower incomes proportionally more (McKenna et al., 2017). In a taxation model the relative contribution of other funding sources can fluctuate over time. In the UK for example, the contribution drawn from user charges has been as high as 5% in 1960, to 1.2% between 2007 and 2011 (Hawe & Cockcroft, 2013, cited by McKenna et al., 2017). The uptake of private healthcare insurance currently stands at 10.6% of the population.

As with many countries worldwide political debate drives the UK government to secure the best health outcomes for the population, while operating within a relatively stable taxation-based model for financing/funding healthcare. However, the tension between an appeal to the majority of the electorate on the one hand, and the increasing cost of providing fundamentally free healthcare to an ageing population on the other, has seen the NHS experiencing the longest and most severe slowdown in funding in its history, thus raising questions about the sustainability of the current funding model (McKenna et al., 2017).

The Impact of the EU Referendum on Healthcare in the UK

The impact of the UK's vote to leave the EU could have major implications for health and social care not least because it has ushered in a period of significant economic and politic uncertainty at a time when the health and care system is already facing huge operational and financial pressures (McKenna, 2016). While the ramifications of the vote remain unclear nevertheless it is expected to affect staffing levels, access to treatment both here and abroad, regulation pertaining to the nursing (and medical) profession, cross boarder cooperation, and funding and finance. The UK currently provides most treatments free of charge for its residents. However, the financial realities of doing so impact the ability of the NHS to upgrade its services and to devote resources to research and development. The decision to leave the EU, may significantly impact health and social care, especially if the UK enters a technical recession.

Organisation of Healthcare in the UK

In the UK healthcare, has been separated into two broad functions, those dealing with medical/clinical care or provision of healthcare services, and those dealing with strategy and policy making and management. Medical and clinical services are subdivided into primary care (community services, general practitioner (GP) services, dentistry and pharmacy services), secondary care (hospital care through referral from GPs), and tertiary care (specialist hospitals). However, the distinction between these two broad functions has become increasingly blurred, which has reflected a general shift in thinking around healthcare with a move towards more local decision-making, removal of barriers between primary and secondary care and more emphasis on patient choice (see Grosios, Gahan, & Burbidge, 2010, pp. 529–534 and Britnell, 2015, pp. 121–128, for a full discussion of UK health services). Responsibility for healthcare and health policy in England currently remains with central government, whereas in Scotland, Wales and Northern Ireland the responsibility for determining both health policy and health services lies with the respective devolved governments. In light of the decision to leave the EU, and subsequent call for a second referendum on an independent Scotland it remains to be seen how health services will be funded and organised across the UK in the future.

The National Health Service

The NHS, as most are aware, came into existence on the 5th July 1948, in the aftermath of World War II, following a proposal to Parliament within the 1942 Beveridge report on Social Insurance and Allied Services. The founding principles of the NHS are credited to Aneurin Bevan, then Minister of Health and have come to determine how we think about health services in the UK, and indeed what we have come to expect. Consequently, any attempt over the decades since 1948 to change the fundamental manner in which our health services are funded and delivered continues to be met with opposition from political parties, activists and think tanks, as well as from an electorate who remain, for the most part, committed to principles of universality, healthcare free at the point of delivery, equity and healthcare paid for by central funding (Grosios et al., 2010). The NHS as we experience it today is made up of a complex range of organisations with different functions and responsibilities (McKenna et al., 2017), which derive from the major changes to the structure of health services in England enshrined within the Health and Social Care Act of 2012. The aim of the Act was to create a greater separation between the Secretary of State for Health and the Department of Health on the one hand and the routine provision of NHS services on the other. Government funding for the NHS is transferred from the Department of Health (around £95 billion each year) to NHS England, an independent body accountable to the Secretary of State, which then allocates most of this money to around 200 clinical commissioning groups (CCGs). CCGs commission or buy care for their populations from providers, which may be run directly by the NHS or by private or third sector organisations (McKenna et al., 2017). NHS England may also directly purchase specialist services and primary care services, for example GP practices, although Mckenna et al. (2017) point out this function may move at some point to the CCGs. Despite relatively consistent funding arrangements over time, a central criticism of the NHS is the historic and continued separation of healthcare from social care. The impact of an ageing population with long-term health conditions and co-morbidities, coupled with the escalating cost of healthcare requires government, now more than ever, to address the concern for a better integrated health and social care system, and it is this that is driving recent government efforts to reform the NHS.

The Five Year Forward View

In 2014, NHS England published the 'Five Year Forward View' which set out a plan to change the way services operate in order to deliver better care with less resource. The plan acknowledges the NHS has dramatically improved over the last 15 years but states there is much still to do. Quality of care is said to be variable, preventable illness widespread and health inequalities deep-rooted (NHS England, 2014, p. 4). The plan recognises that patients' needs are changing, and new treatment options are emerging. Particular challenges are said to include areas such as mental health, cancer and support for frail older patients.

Against this backdrop, NHS England makes the case for further reform to an NHS which has already witnessed the most radical reforms since its inception in 1948. The Five Year Forward View claims a broad consensus exists about the way forward for the NHS, which should include a radical upgrade of prevention and public health, greater control for patients over their own care, and decisive steps to break down the barriers between how care is provided, that is, better integration of services including those between health and social care. These ideas are not new. Indeed, a major criticism of the NHS over the decades since its inception has been the lack of vision for the integration of health and social care. What is new though is the suggestion for an eclectic approach to the delivery of services. NHS England provides a rationale for eclecticism in that in a diverse England a 'one size fits all' care model will not work, while at the same time nor is the answer to let a 'thousand flowers bloom' (NHS

England, 2014, p. 5). It follows logically for the plan to suggest new options including multispecialty community provider schemes whereby groups of GPs combine with nurses, other community health services, hospital specialists, and possibly with mental health and social care to create integrated out-of-hospital care, and integrated hospital and primary care services, which combine general practice and hospital services.

Further reforms to the NHS include the redesigning of non-urgent and emergency care in order to integrate accident and emergency (A&E) departments, GP out-of-hours services, urgent care centres, NHS 111 and ambulance services. These reforms, say NHS England, will require strong national leadership and meaningful local flexibility in the way payment rules, regulatory requirements and other mechanisms are applied. Worrying, the Five Year Forward View then makes a commitment to investing in new options for the NHS workforce, raising the game on health technology, investing in research and innovation and developing new 'test bed' sites for worldwide innovators, and new 'green field' sites where completely new NHS services will be designed from scratch (p. 6). And all this at a time when the NHS is quite possibly in its worst financial position in its history.

Since publication of the Five Year Forward View, in spite of its positive rhetoric, evidence suggests a less optimistic picture. In its report on progress on NHS Reform, the independent non-party think tank *Reform* suggest that while savings have been made through short-term efficiencies and not sustainable reform to services, when looking across the NHS, there has been disappointing progress towards a more sustainable workforce, a more integrated health service, greater capacity in out-of-hospital care, greater use of alternatives to A&E, and greater competition and patient choice (Corrie & Mosseri-Marlio, 2015, p. 5). To summarise, NHS hospital deficits were expected to total £800 million in 2014/2015, with an additional £2 billion in funding required compared to the settlement of 2010. In reality, NHS providers in England ended 2015–2016 with a deficit of £2.45 billion, which is the second year in succession whereby the NHS has ended in the red, thus raising concerns that spending limits placed on the Department of Health's spending limit will be breached (Dunn, McKenna, and Murray, 2016). It seems fair to say that recent reforms have not, so far at least, achieved the desired outcomes as stated in NHS England's Five Year Forward View. In spite of unprecedented increases in funding over the last decade, and with little evidence that radical overhaul and reform has brought about the desired outcomes, it is against this backdrop that the first hospital has been put into special administration.

Mid Staffordshire NHS Foundation Trust

Every nurse and midwife practising in the UK today, most members of the general public, and, no doubt, a good deal of people working in health and care settings across the globe will know something about Mid Staffordshire (NHS) Foundation Hospital Trust (MSFT). The 'scandal' as it has come to be known, surrounding MSFT arose from a 'disputed' claim that between 400 and 1200 patients died as a result of poor care over the 50 months between January 2005 and March 2009 at Stafford hospital, a small district general hospital in Staffordshire. The hospital, which has since been renamed the County Hospital was run by MSFT and supervised by West Midlands Strategic Health Authority. Following concerns about high mortality rates at the hospital coupled with a growing number of complaints from patients and those close to them who had experienced exceedingly poor care whilst at the hospital a non-statutory inquiry was commissioned and subsequently led by The Secretary of State for Health, the Right Honourable Andy Burnham MP, in July 2009.

The inquiry culminating in the Francis Report in 2013 changed the face of healthcare in the UK and has been widely reported, commented on, discussed and written about by almost everyone with an interest in healthcare, from politicians, the media, healthcare professionals, academics, and the public. The events surrounding MSFT were catastrophic and led to what can fairly be described as an apocalypse in healthcare in the UK, that is, of such magnitude as to define healthcare in terms of before and after (pre- and post) Francis. All stakeholders in healthcare have a legitimate right to be concerned about what happened at Stafford District Hospital, of this there is no doubt. However, some stakeholders have clearly taken what happened at MSFT to support a political agenda aimed at reforming healthcare services along particular ideological lines.

Evidence for this lies in the complete misuse of Hospital Standardised Mortality Ratios (HSMR) to suggest Stafford District Hospital was performing far worse than other similar hospitals, when in fact the method used to analyse HSMR data (the Doctor Foster method) has been shown to exhibit methodological bias, be open to coding errors, and is not a credible method for claiming variation in mortality ratios reflects differences in quality of care (Walker, 2013).

What is clear though is the management of the hospital became dominated by financial pressures and achieving Foundation Trust status, to the detriment of quality of care and many patients suffered greatly as a result (Francis, 2013). So why did MSFT become so focused on achieving Foundation Trust Status to the clear detriment of patient care. To answer this question, we need to look at the reasons behind this ideological shift in thinking around how hospitals, which up to this point had been historically managed within the framework of the NHS, could be better managed.

NHS Foundation Trusts are not-for profit public benefit corporations created to devolve decision-making about a hospitals healthcare provision away from central government to local organisations and communities. Freedom from Whitehall is key in order for Foundation Trusts, not directed by government, to have a greater freedom to decide with their governors and members their own strategy and how services are run. Foundation Trusts can retain their surpluses and can borrow to invest in services for patients and service users. Foundation Trusts are accountable through their governors and members to local communities, to their commissioners through contracts, and to Parliament, the CQC, and to Monitor. Monitor is an executive non-departmental public body sponsored by the Department of Health to act as the sector regulator for health services in England. Its job is essentially to make the health sector work better for patients. It does this by 'monitoring' how public sector healthcare provider services are being led, by ensuring NHS services continue if a healthcare provider is in difficulty, ensuring the NHS payment system rewards quality and efficiency, and that choice and quality operate in the best interests of patients and service users.

The idea of hospitals as Foundation Trusts is credited to Alan Milburn who, as Labour's Health Secretary in 2002, announced a plan to allow the private sector to take over management of England's failing hospitals. The rationale behind the creation of Foundation Trusts was for hospitals who had consistently failed to raise standards to franchise management of the hospital to either another public-sector health organisation or, in time, a not-for profit organisation such as a university of charity. The hospitals assets were to remain in public ownership. While Alan Milburn stressed the creation of Foundation Trusts was not a closet move to privatise the NHS, many commentators at the time believed the move represented just that. David Hinchliffe, Chairman of the House of Commons Health Select Committee, found the creation of franchises incredibly worrying and felt that the Labour government's policy was beginning to resemble that of the previous Conservative government.

In spite of criticism and concern over what appeared to be a move towards privatisation of the NHS, a claim hotly disputed by Alan Milburn, the first wave of ten hospitals became Trusts in 2004. Successive governments have set dates by which all NHS Trusts were to achieve Foundation Trust status and in 2011 the Health and Social Care Bill proposed that all NHS Trusts become Foundation Trusts. However, it soon became clear a significant number of NHS Trusts would never become Foundation Trusts. To address the dissonance between rhetoric and reality the NHS Trust Development Authority was established through the Health and Social Care Act (2012) with a remit to supervise Trusts who have not achieved Foundation Trust Status. In 2016, of 247 providers of acute, mental health and community NHS services, 157 are Foundation Trusts, whose performance is reported on by Monitor (GOV.UK, 2016).

When concerns are raised about the quality of care hospitals are delivering, they can be put into 'special measures'. Special measures offer hospital trusts the support deemed necessary in order for them to improve performance, in addition to giving the public the ability to hold hospital trusts to account (GOV.UK, 2016). 'NHS Improvement' supports foundation trusts to give patients consistently safe, high-quality, compassionate care within local health systems that are financially sustainable and is the operational name for the organisation, which brings together Monitor, the NHS Trust Development Authority, Patient Safety, the National Reporting and Learning System, the Advancing Change Team, and the Intensive Support Teams, all of whom have a designated role in monitoring, supporting and improving the performance of hospital trusts, and taking action when trusts are deemed to be failing. Hospital trusts can be placed into special measures on recommendation from the Chief Inspector of Hospitals, currently Sir Mike Richards, after a routine inspection. The Chief Inspector of Hospitals acts on behalf of the CQC, the body charged with monitoring, inspecting and regulating healthcare services to ensure fundamental standards of safety and quality are being met. CQC publish their findings, including performance ratings in a bid to assist the public to choose care (CQC, 2016).

Once a hospital trust has been placed into special measures a series of actions are triggered, typically including:

- Partnership with a high-performing NHS foundation trust or NHS trust to help deliver improvements
- Requirement for the trust to produce a regularly updated action plan, published on the NHS Choices website, and detailing progress towards improvement
- The appointment of an improvement director—appointed by and accountable to NHS Improvement
- Possible suspension of some of the additional freedoms integral to foundation trust status, for example freedom to act as an autonomous body, to appoint executive teams and determine operating plans
- Review of leadership, with subsequent changes to management teams to ensure best leadership in order to drive forward improvements in an efficient and timely fashion.

The approach of the current Conservative government towards apparently 'failing' foundation hospital trusts is punitive, disciplinary and correctional. Putting a hospital trust into special measures, serves as both a label of failure, an act of public scrutiny, and a notice served to 'do better'. In the words of the Jeremy Hunt, Secretary of State for Health:

> Turning special measures hospitals round is my top priority as Health Secretary. For too long, patients have had to put up with poor care because it was inconvenient to expose and tackle failure. So today I am committing

to total transparency on progress in these hospitals and to leave no stone unturned in our mission to turn them round (Hunt, 2013).

Monitor, which became part of NHS Improvement from 1st April 2016, reports on the performance of NHS foundation trust hospitals using two ratings. The 'financial sustainability' risk rating is Monitor's view of the level of financial risk a foundation trust faces and its overall financial efficiency. Foundation trusts can be rated from 1 as the most serious risk to 4, as the least risk. A rating of 2* means the trust has a risk rating of 2, but its financial position is considered unlikely to worsen in the immediate future. The 'governance' rating is Monitor's degree of concern as to how a trust is run. Monitor report this rating in terms of 'no evident concerns', 'enforcement action begun' or that a trust is 'under review' (concerns identified, but no action yet taken). In June 2016, Monitor reported on the financial sustainability and governance of 157 hospital foundation trusts. Seventy-one (45%) were given a financial sustainability risk rating of 2. The fact that none of the 71 received a rating of 2* is suggestive that the financial position of these trusts is set to worsen. Monitor rated 19 (12%) trusts at level 1, most serious risk, with 33 trusts (21%) at level 4, or least risk. No data were reported for four trusts. In terms of governance, which Monitor categorise using a simplified traffic light system, 85 (54%) received a green rating, or no evident concerns. However, 42 (26%) trusts received a red rating and subject to enforcement action, 6 (14%) of which were put into special measures. A further 26 trusts of the total 157 were requested to provide Monitor with more information following apparent multiple breaches in achieving various targets, for example A&E waiting times, or cancer targets, or following a deterioration in the trusts financial position. These figures clearly depict a worsening crisis, both in terms of financial sustainability and governance with the NHS in England. Among the most punitive measures towards improving quality and efficiency within NHS hospitals is the perverse incentivising of high-performing trusts, who are able to enter a contractual arrangement with the NHS Trust Authority to support hospital trusts in special measures. These so-called high-performing trusts have access to a special incentive fund, through which, where appropriate, they could be paid extra, if they help produce real results (GOV.UK,

2016). In essence, what this means is that underperforming hospital trusts are unlikely to benefit from much needed extra resources, in spite of the fact that most of the trusts receiving a red rating, that is, giving cause for concern within Monitor's reporting framework, also received a financial sustainability risk rating of 2 or less, while, with few exceptions, the trusts receiving a green governance rating, or 'no evident concerns' were the same trusts receiving a financial sustainability risk rating of 3 or more, or 'at least risk'. Ironically the financially viable high-performing trusts are incentivised through access to a special fund at the expense of finically struggling underperforming trusts.

Replacing the old approach of paying management consultants to analyse the problems of underperforming hospitals by giving contracts to 'the best' in the NHS has not seen the success envisioned by the Secretary of State for Health in his press release in 2013. However, Dr Mark Porter, Chair of the British Medical Association, suggests the governments pursuit of a fuller seven-day NHS in England through the imposition of new pay and working arrangements for junior doctors has served to focus attention away from the huge financial problems of the NHS and onto a corrosive dispute on a principle on which doctors fundamentally agree.

Next Steps on the Five Year Forward View

In March 2017, NHS England published The Next Steps on the Five Year Forward View. The document reviews the progress made since the launch of the original plans in October 2014, before setting out a series of steps for the NHS to deliver a more responsive and better organised NHS in England. In the document, Simon Stevens, CEO of NHS England draws attention to the availability of new treatments for a growing and ageing population, which have placed more pressure on the service than ever before. Nevertheless, treatment outcomes are reported to be far better, with public satisfaction with the NHS said to be higher than 10 or 20 years ago (NHS England, 2017). The point of the publication though is not to simply update on progress made in the areas laid out in the original document, but to set out how the NHS needs to adapt to take advantage of the opportunities that science and technology offers to patients, carers and those who serve them, and to evolve to meet new challenges brought about by an ageing population with complex health issues. However, while the government appears to be setting out plans to ensure the NHS, which continues to matter to the public, can deliver high-quality healthcare, in reality, funding for the NHS is in serious decline, and has not kept pace with average health spending in the 14 other countries of the EU. While comparing healthcare spending between countries is not straightforward, nevertheless John Appleby, former Chief Economist at the King's Fund, points to the differences in the source of funding, public or private, which need to be considered when making comparisons, and suggests it is usual to compare total spending (public plus private) expressed as a proportion of countries' gross domestic product (GDP). He concludes, on this basis, using Organisation for Economic Co-operation and Development data, that in 2013 the UK spent 8.5% of its GDP on public and private healthcare, which placed the UK 13th out of the original 15 countries of the EU, and 1.7 percentage points lower than the EU-14's level of spending (Appleby, 2016). The continued chronic underfunding of healthcare in the UK, despite government rhetoric is exacerbated by the UK's vote to leave the EU, which is likely to have major implications for health and social care, not least because it has ushered in a period of significant economic and political uncertainty at a time when the health and care system is facing major operational and financial pressures. McKenna (2016) points to five big issues for health and social care after the Brexit vote, including staffing, accessing treatment abroad, regulation, cross-border cooperation, and funding and finance. She concludes the Department of Health now faces the massive task of reviewing individual EU regulations and deciding whether each one should be repealed or replaced with UK-drafted alternatives. Like other government departments, the Department of Health faces significant capacity issues as it is currently implementing a programme to reduce the number of staff in the Department by about one-third over the course of this parliament. In addition to work generated by the Brexit vote, the Department of Health faces a back log of policy announcements and publications, which were held in abeyance during the referendum period, some of which may not be published. While the immediate attention surrounding Brexit has not prevented the publication of the Next Steps on the Five Year Forward View, nevertheless the financial ramifications of Brexit on health and social care spending will not be known for some time to come. With regard to the persistent difficulties concerning how best to manage and subsequently fund the integration of health and social care the Next Steps on the Five Year Forward View refers to the original publication, which stated;

> The traditional divide between primary care, community services, and hospitals—largely unaltered since the birth of the NHS—is increasingly a barrier to the personalised and coordinated health services patients need…. (NHS England, 2014)

The updated strategy highlights the progress made on the original plans, in particular the Vanguard Programme, in which 50 areas around England covering more than five million people worked to redesign care through a focus on better integration of community services in combination with joined up health services (NHS England, 2017). Of these 50 original geographical areas, 29 were subsequently chosen to develop new models of care under the 'new care models programme'. The vanguards, as these areas became known, are partnerships of NHS, local government, voluntary, community and other organisations that are implementing plans to improve the healthcare people receive, prevent ill health and save funds. However, implementation of 'Vanguard' has been beset with challenges, not least organisational issues, communication difficulties between Vanguard and non-Vanguard areas, development needs of staff and difficulties in achieving collective belief in the Vanguard programme. Clearly, 'Vanguard' is envisaged as a comprehensive change programme, designed to address the serious efficiency gap within the NHS over the next few years. However, the day to day challenge of joining up health and social care for patients with complex care needs continues to prove immensely challenging for the NHS and led to the publication of more planning guidance in the shape of Sustainability and Transformation Plans (STPs).

Sustainability and Transformation Plans

STPs cover all aspects of spending in the NHS in England for a period of five years (October, 2016 to March 2021). Forty-four areas with an average population of 1.2 million people were originally identified as the 'geographical footprints on which the plans were based'. The development of STPs has been led by a named experienced professional, for the most part drawn from CCGs or from NHS hospital trusts, although some have come from local government. While the broad scope of STPs is to improve quality and to develop new models of care, improve health and well-being, and to improve efficiency of services, nevertheless a number of concerns have been raised regarding implementation of the plans. A shortage of cash to kick start change, too little progress on a payment system which encourages collaboration, the need to sort out the debacle of the contracting rules, which emerged from the Lansley reforms and rushing change have all been cited as hampering progress (Ham cited by Vize, 2016).

While much effort has been expended over time to address the organisational and financial challenges of integrating health and social care, nevertheless it remains the optimum solution to the increasing cost of providing universal healthcare in the context of an ageing population with complex care needs. The challenge for the NHS, the social care and the voluntary sector is to focus less on the question of what is the matter *with* the patient, and to focus more on the question of what matters *to* the patient. Reframing questions around the integration of health and social care in this way opens up new possibilities for rethinking health and social care services, which more fully reflect the centrality of the service user in decisions concerning treatment and care, thus releasing the potential for co-productive approaches to service planning, design and delivery.

Co-Production in Healthcare: An Alternative Approach

The apparent failure of successive governments, since the inception of the NHS in 1948, to reform health service delivery mechanisms has given rise to a new conversation, which argues that the key to reforming public services is to encourage users to design and deliver services in equal partnership with professionals: in other words, co-production, as a different way of 'doing care and support' (Carr, 2014). The origins of co-production can be traced back to the USA in the 1970s when the political economist Elinor Ostrom and colleagues became disillusioned with increasingly centralised and bureaucratised police services. Ostrom and colleagues developed the term co-production to describe relationships, which could potentially exist between, what they called the 'regular' producer (street-level police officers, school teachers or health workers) and 'clients', who want to be transformed by the service into safer, better educated or healthier people (Ostrom, 1996). The notion of co-production was later built on by Edgar Cahn, a civil rights lawyer and legal academic, who drew on the concept as a means of developing the 'core economy', which he argued meant using the resources embedded in people's everyday lives and relationships, such as loyalty, vigilance, empathy, love, understanding, trust, knowledge, experience and skills. Co-production, in the sense of the core economy facilitates a definition of productivity, which takes account of social, as well as economic contributors. Cahn's notion of co-production is contextualised as being about valuing all human capacity, honouring all contributions, and generating reciprocity (Cahn, 2004). Resurgence of interest in co-production relates to a continued and growing concern that reform of public services, including health services has failed to address an unprecedented set of challenges, including increasing demand for services, rising expectation, seemingly intractable social problems and, in many cases, reduced budgets (Boyle & Harris, 2009). With respect to a delivery model for health services co-production is thought to offer solutions particularly for the sharing of information, and on shared decision-making between service users and providers (Betancourt, Ostrom, Brown, & Roundtree, 2002; Needham & Carr, 2002).

The principles of co-production are transferable to any situation involving relationships between users of a service and providers of services, being most often associated with mental health and social care. With regard to healthcare, co-production has been discussed particularly with respect to models of service delivery for clients with long-term health conditions, examples of which include the expert patient programme. The core values and principles underpinning co-production, determined by Cahn (2004) and cited by Carr (2014) in the 'Guide to co-production in mental health and social care' require the following:

- An asset perspective: 'no more throwaway people'
- Redefining work: 'no more taking the social contribution of people for granted'
- Reciprocity: 'stop creating dependencies and devaluing those whom you help while you profit from their troubles'
- Social capital: 'no more disinvesting in families; neighbourhoods and communities'

When using the core values as a baseline Edgar Cahn was able to map out what co-production means on both individual and societal levels. At the level of the individual co-production enables recognition that everyone needs to be needed regardless of age, formal credentials, marketable skills or barriers. Co-production entails the fulfilment of that need where one's contribution is acknowledged, recorded and extremely validated (Cahn, 2004). It necessarily follows that seeking support does not result in dependence, but rather interdependence.

Co-production is premised on the view that individuals are embedded in social contexts. For societal co-production Cahn, cited by Carr (2014, p. 3) sees a "shift in relationships between professionals and service users/communities, which moves from one of subordination and dependency to parity, mutuality and reciprocity". In this sense important philosophical and pragmatic lessons can be drawn from co-production values and principles for nursing and nurse education, which suffer from subordination and dependency on a number of levels; subordination of nursing to the medical profession, subordination of nurse education to the nursing profession, subordination of nurse education by the government, and dependency of nurse education on the regulatory and oversight functions of the professional body, the NMC. Co-production, with its emphasis on a framework of participation, collaborative processes, a set of standards based on an asset perspective, and a redefining of work, reciprocity and social capital, provides a useful basis for critical conversations concerned with transforming nurse education, together with political, organisational and socially oriented conversations around transformation of health and social care. Co-production and its place in nurse education is discussed more fully in Chap. 5.

Nursing and Nurse Education After Francis

The Francis Inquiry marked a turning point in the recent history of the NHS. Fundamental questions were asked about the multiple cultures, values, aims, expectations, disciplines and practices of hundreds of national, regional and local organisations within an NHS, which was deemed to be no longer a unified system. The ensuing report made 290 recommendations, to different parts of the NHS, including healthcare regulators, providers and government. A key recommendation included the introduction of a new statutory 'Duty of Candour', which places a legal obligation on NHS organisations and individual practitioners to be honest and truthful in all their dealings with patients and the public. This duty of candour is arguably a direct response to the claim by relatives of patients; in total 164 witnesses gave evidence at the inquiry, of the dismissive way in which their enquires were treated.

Candour places a duty on healthcare professionals, in all care settings, to tell a patient when something has gone wrong, to try and put things right, and to apologise. However, this duty of candour is not new for medical professionals, or indeed for nurses.

The General Medical Council clarified its position on candour in 1998 when it introduced an ethical obligation for medical professionals to be open and honest when things go wrong. Similarly, the NMC requires nurses to be open and candid with all service users about all aspects of care and treatment, including when any mistakes or harm have taken place. The Code: Professional standards of practice and behaviour for nurses and midwives (NMC, 2015b) specifically requires nurses and midwives to act immediately to put right the situation if someone has suffered actual harm for any reason or an incident has happened which had the potential for harm, explain fully and promptly what has happened, including the likely effects and apologise to the person affected and where appropriate, their advocate, family or carers, and to document all events formally and take further action if appropriate, so that issues can be dealt with quickly. The duty of candour, introduced by government on the 1st April, 2013 applies to contracts for NHS and non-NHS providers of services to NHS patients. It does not apply to services commissioned under primary care contracts, or to many private providers, which leaves open the question of whether the private sector is considered by government to provide better healthcare and therefore should be less subject to regulation.

The duty of candour only applies to the most serious injuries, defined as moderate, severe injury or death, which again begs the question as to whether government views smaller injuries or those considered less moderate as not deserving of explanation or apology (Malsher, 2013). Given the potential for the stressful working conditions reported by the Royal College of Nursing (RCN) to continue, including heavy workloads, staff shortages, frustrations with paperwork, targets and a lack of resources such as equipment and IT (RCN, 2013b), the question remains as to whether the imposition of a statutory duty of candour will impact the likelihood that mistakes made by healthcare professionals will be acknowledged and reported on.

With respect to the RCN, the Francis Report heavily criticised the role of the College, suggesting it should have done more to support its members on the ground. The report thus recommended the RCN split its employee function, that is, its function as a trade union, from its professional function. However, this recommendation garnered little support from its membership who overwhelmingly expressed the view that the College should maintain its structure, as the relationship between the trade union function and professional function make for a stronger organisation. With particular reference to nurse education the RCN have called into question the recommendation for recruitment of student nurses who exhibit the right values, display a desire to deliver compassionate care and learn the technical skills essential to modern day nursing. These recommendations appeared to assume student nurses, at the time of the inquiry at least, did not exhibit the right values, display a desire to deliver compassionate care and learn the technical skills essential to modern day nurses.

The Francis Report called for a national entry-level requirement that nursing students spend a minimum period of time, at least three months, working on the direct care of patients under the supervision of a registered nurse. Again, this recommendation was challenged by the RCN in that it seems not to recognise the extent of the practical experience currently undertaken by nursing students on programmes whereby 50% of time is spent in clinical practice (for a comprehensive response to the recommendations directed at nursing and nurse education see RCN, 2013b Mid Staffordshire NHS Foundation Trust Public Inquiry Report: response of the Royal College of Nursing at www.rcn.org.uk).

Prior to publication of the Francis Report, in the face of concerns of poor nursing care, which imply the quality of initial nursing education is at fault, the RCN commissioned its own independent review. The Willis Commission on Nursing Education, launched in April 2012 under the chairmanship of Lord Willis of Knaresborough, had a remit to establish what excellent nursing education in the UK should look like and how it should be delivered. The Commission specifically asked:

> What essential features of pre-registration nursing education in the UK, and what types of support for newly registered practitioners, are needed to create and maintain a workforce of competent, compassionate nurses fit to deliver future health and social care services?

Among its key recommendations, the Willis Commission advised nurse education programmes should be better evaluated, and based on extensive research in order to provide evidence of correlations between current practice, entry criteria and selection processes, attrition rates and course outcomes. No mention is made of pedagogical research to underpin nurse education programmes, in spite of recommendations for programme content to foster professionalism, for patient-centred care to be a golden thread running through programmes, and for universities to value nursing as a practice and research discipline. The RCN, in countering criticisms of nurse education, point to the Willis Commission, which found no evidence of shortcomings in nurse education which could be directly responsible for poor standards of care or a decline in care standards (Willis Commission, 2012).

Unlike the NMC whereby the Council's regulatory function has severely impacted the capacity for nurse educationalists to determine appropriate and innovative pedagogy for nurse education in the twenty-first century, the RCN appears cognisant of the need for alternative pedagogical solutions for nurse education. The RCN, while not directly discussing pedagogy, quote the Council of Deans of Health, who see students as a catalyst for change: part of the solution not the problem (RCN, 2013b). Such student-centred pedagogies, whose central tenet is to develop learner autonomy, independence, skills and practices that enable lifelong learning and independent problem-solving, are more likely to lead to the type of nurse envisioned by Sir Robert Francis, as opposed to over regulation, ever more rigorous application of standards, and ill thought out requirements for entry into a profession already suffering from under recruitment of UK trained nurses. In short, positivist solutions continued to be proposed to the detriment of innovative pedagogical curriculum development. This lack of attention to student-centred pedagogy is not confined to the micro level of programmes, but is in fact evidence of a more far reaching concerns. Stiegler (2015) notes that contemporary universities are inculcating the very conditions of stupidity, by which he means that embedding universities in global neoliberal economies leads to an uncritical acceptance of knowledge handed down prescriptively, and to the claims that there is no alternative, or that things "have to be this way". Increasingly the struggle to help students towards an academic maturity in which they are knowledgeable about their discipline, but have had nurtured the critical capacity to develop, contest and create alternative visions, is eroded. Such developments in the UK are exemplified in proposals for a Teaching Excellence Framework, whose principal components of measurement (student satisfaction, employment rates and salary levels) are arguably invalid assessments of the quality of teaching. Increasingly, argues Stiegler (2015), the freedom to learn (in the sense of inculcating deep attention in students) is located in spaces outside the neoliberal university, and the challenge for a critical pedagogy is how to make links to such new communities of learning. Volunteering and reflecting upon activities supporting marginalised communities may be one way of reclaiming critical insight for the nursing curriculum.

Conclusion

This chapter has set the scene for a discussion of innovative and transformative pedagogy for nurse education, as an appropriate response to the criticism and ensuing debate around nursing and nurse education, in the aftermath of the Francis Inquiry into failings at Mid Staffordshire NHS Foundation Trust. The current context of healthcare services is argued to severely impact the capacity for nurses to think creatively, and to arrive at solutions to problems of finite resources, staff shortages, and rising public expectation in terms of diagnosis, treatment, and acute and long-term care. The imposition of a duty of candour, whereby healthcare professionals have a responsibility to acknowledge and report when care falls below acceptable standards is unlikely to impact quality of care, if nursing curricula continues to inadequately prepare nurses for contemporary nursing practice. Critical pedagogy is postulated as a means to address the challenges facing nurse education in the post-Francis era. The concept of co-production was suggested as an antidote to perceived failures to reform healthcare services along New Public Management lines, which is argued to lead to punitive, disciplinary and correctional measures. Co-production is recognised as a potential framework for engaging stakeholders in critical conversations around the transformation of nurse education, in addition to transformation of healthcare services. Co-production has, at its foundation, an 'asset' perspective, recognition of the social contribution of people, collaboration, cooperation and recognition that confrontation, in particular in relation to circumstances of social injustice is a necessary attribute of professional nursing practice. In this sense, co-production is congruent with the philosophical underpinnings of critical pedagogy, which attempts to help students to question and challenge posited domination and to undermine the beliefs and practices that are alleged to dominate (Freire, 1972).

The following chapter discusses global health, standards for global nurse education and global standards for the preparation of nurse educators. Consideration is given to the World Health Organisation's efforts to address complexities in healthcare provision, health professionals at different levels, and the need to assure more equitable access to healthcare through standardisation of nurse education and nurse educator programmes. The impact of standardisation of initial nurse education on an increasingly migratory nursing workforce is analysed.

References

Appleby, J. (2016). How does NHS spending compare with health spending internationally? Retrieved April 24, 2017, from https://www.kingsfund.org.uk/blog/2016/01/how-does-nhs-spending-compare-health-spending-internationally

Betancourt, L. A., Ostrom, A. L., Brown, S. W., & Roundtree, R. I. (2002). Client co-production in knowledge-intensive business services. *California Management Review, 44*, 100–128.

Boyle, D., & Harris, M. (2009). *The challenge of co-production: How equal partnerships between professionals and the public are crucial to improving public services*. Discussion paper, NESTA, London.

Britnell, M. (2015). *In search of the perfect health system*. London: Palgrave Macmillan.

Cahn, E. S. (2004). *No more throw-away people: The co-production imperative* (1st ed.). Washington, DC: Essential Books.

Carr, S. (2014). *Guide to co-production in mental health and social care*. Community Care Inform Adults (online resource).

Cooper, Z., Gibbon, S., Jones, S., & McGuire, A. (2011). Does hospital competition save lives? Evidence from the English NHS patient choice reforms. *The Economic Journal, 121*(554), F228–F260.

Corrie, C., & Mosseri-Marlio, W. (2015). *Progress on NHS reform*. London: Reform.

Council for Healthcare and Regulatory Excellence. (2012). *Strategic review of the nursing and midwifery council: Final report*. London: CHRE.

Council of Deans of Health. (2016). Educating the future nurse – A paper for discussion. Retrieved November 9, 2016, from www.councilofdeans.org.uk

CQC. (2016). Retrieved from http://www.cqc.org.uk/content/special-measures

Dunn, P., McKenna, H., & Murray, R. (2016). Deficits in the NHS 2016. https://www.kingsfund.org.uk/publications/deficits-nhs-2016?

Dyson, S. E., Liu, L. Q., van den Akker, O., & O'Driscoll, M. (2017). The extent, variability and attitudes towards volunteering among undergraduate nursing students: Implications for pedagogy in nurse education. *Nurse Education in Practice, 23*, 15–22.

Escotet, M. A. (2012). *There is today a need to educate for uncertainty.* The Escotet Foundation. Retrieved June 5, 2016, from http://escotet.org/2014/01/today-there-is-a-need-to-educate-for-uncertainty/

Francis, R. (2013). *Report of the Mid Staffordshire NHS Foundation Trust public inquiry.* London: The Stationery Office.

Freire, P. (1972). *Pedagogy of the oppressed.* London: Penguin Books.

Gov.UK. (2016). Transparency data: NHS foundation trust directory. Retrieved from https://www.gov.uk/government/publications/nhs-foundation-trust-directory/nhs-foundation-trust-directory

Grosios, K., Gahan, P. B., & Burbidge, J. (2010). Overview of healthcare in the UK. *The EPMA Journal, 1*(4), 529–534.

Hawe, E., & Cockcroft, L. (2013). *OHE guide to health and health care statistics* (2nd ed.). London: Office of Health Economics.

Health and Social Care Information Centre. (2016). Prescriptions dispensed in the community: England 2005–2015 (online). NHS Digital website. Retrieved August 8, 2017, from http://content.digital.nhs.uk/catalogue/PUB20664

Hughes, R. G. (2008). Nurses at the "sharp end" of patient care. In R. G. Hughes (Ed.), *Patient safety and quality: An evidence-based handbook for nurses.* Rockville, MD: AHRQ Publishers.

Hunt. (2013). Cited in Department of Health press release. Hunt sets out tough new to turn around NHS hospitals. Retrieved from https://www.gov.uk/government/news/hunt-sets-out-tough-new-approach-to-turn-around-nhs-hospitals

Ironside, P. M. (2001). Creating a research base for nursing education: An interpretive review of conventional, critical, feminist, postmodern, and phenomenologic pedagogies. *Advances in Nursing Science, 23*(3), 72–87.

Macleod Clark, J. (2016). *Developing new standards for the future graduate registered nurse.* Council of Deans. Retrieved April 25, 2017, from https://councilofdeans.org.uk/2016/08/developing-new-standards-for-the-future-graduate-registered-nurse/

Malsher, A. (2013). Duty of candour: Patients deserve more protection than simple contracts. Retrieved from https://www.theguardian.com/healthcare-network/2013/apr/03/nhs-reforms-duty-of-candour-mid-staffs-scandal

McKenna, H. (2016). Five big issues for health and social care after the Brexit vote. Retrieved April 24, 2017, from https://www.kingsfund.org.uk/publications/articles/brexit-and-nhs

McKenna, H., Dunn, P., Northern, E., & Buckley, T. (2017). How health care is funded. *The King's Fund*. Retrieved August 7, 2017, from https://www.kingsfund.org.uk/publications/how-health-care-is-funded

Needham, C., & Carr, S. (2002). SCIE Research Briefing 31: Co-production: An emerging evidence base for adult social care transformation. London: Social Care Institute for Excellence. Retrieved from www.scie.org.co

NHS England. (2014). Five year forward view. Retrieved June 5, 2016, from https://www.england.nhs.uk/wp-content/uploads/2014/10/5yfv-web.pdf

NHS England. (2017). Next steps on the five year forward view. Retrieved April 24, 2017, from https://www.england.nhs.uk/five-year-forward-view/#

NMC. (2015a). *Nursing and midwifery council annual fitness to practise report 2014–2015*, Nursing and Midwifery Council, HMSO, London.

NMC. (2015b). *The code: Professional standards of practice and behaviour for nurses and midwives*. NMC, London. Retrieved from www.nmc-uk.org

NMC. (2016b). *Our role in education*. Retrieved June 5, 2016, from https://www.nmc.org.uk/education/our-role-in-education/

Ostrom, E. (1996). Crossing the great divide: Coproduction, synergy, and development. *World Development, 24*(6), 1073–1087.

PSA. (2014/2015). *Professional standards for authority for health and social care*. Annual Reports and Accounts and Performance Review Report 2014/2015, PSA, London.

RCN. (2013b). *Mid Staffordshire NHS foundation trust: Response of the Royal College of Nursing*. London: RCN. Retrieved from www.rcn.org.uk

Scott, H. (2004). Are nurses too clever to care' and too posh to wash. *British Journal of Nursing, 13*(10), 581.

Stiegler, B. (2015). *States of shock: Stupidity and knowledge in the 21st century: Pharmacology of the university*. Cambridge: Polity Press.

Vize, R. (2016). Sustainability and transformation plans are 'least bad option' for NHS. Retrieved April 25, 2017, from https://www.theguardian.com/healthcare-network/2016/oct/21/sustainability-and-transformation-plans-least-bad-option-nhs

Walker, S. (2013). *Mid Staffs: Was it what we've been told?* Retrieved from https://skwalker1964.wordpress.com/2013/02/26/the-real-mid-staffs-story-one-excess-death-if-that/

Willis Commission. (2012). *Quality with compassion: The future of nursing education*. Report of the Willis Commission, London: RCN. Retrieved from www.williscommission.org.uk

Wittek, L., & Kvernbekk, T. (2011). On the problems of asking for a definition of quality in education. *Scandinavian Journal of Educational Research, 55*(6), 671–684.

3

Global Health and Global Nurse Education

Introduction

This chapter discusses global health services and ways in which nurse education has developed to meet local needs. Factors leading to migration of the nursing workforce are considered with particular reference to the implications of a migratory nursing workforce for nurse education in the UK. The chapter draws on recent evidence around the experience of the overseas nursing workforce in the UK and the implications for practice and education.

The organization of healthcare across the globe is dependent on the wealth of the country under consideration. All industrialised nations, with the exception of the United States implement some form of universal healthcare. The main ways universal healthcare is funded in wealthy nations include government run (tax funded) systems, for example, the NHS; privately run but government pays the lion's share, for example, Canada and France; and private insurance arrangements, with regulation and subsidies to ensure universal coverage and non-discrimination on grounds of medical history and/or pre-existing conditions, for example, Switzerland. In the United States, universal healthcare is not provided for all citizens. Programmes exist for the elderly, military service families, the disabled, children and some poor through Medicare and Medicaid. However, some 45 million people in the United States are currently uninsured, with a further 25 million underinsured (Shah, 2011). In developing countries, that is, those considered not wealthy, while some strive to provide universal healthcare, most struggle to do so, due to lack of resources, inappropriate use of resources or misappropriation of resources to fund war and conflict.

The disparity between nations in healthcare is replicated in approaches to nurse education. For example, the length of nursing programme may vary from 2 to 5 years; some countries offer nursing programmes but no midwifery programmes, some countries see nursing and midwifery as separate professions, while some consider midwifery as an option only for qualified nurses. In 2009, the World Health Organization (WHO) set out to determine global standards for the education of professional nurses and midwives. The WHO global standards are premised on the belief that each country needs to have an adequate and sustainable source of health professionals, trained within the context of current and future issues in patient safety and quality of care (WHO, 2009). While this is a laudable aim in and of itself, the reality is the very countries in most need of highly educated nurses and midwives are likely to be those worse placed to prioritise resources on nursing and midwifery education. These nations suffer most from net migration to wealthy countries where higher standards of living and education are a significant pulling factor in overseas recruitment of nurses and midwives.

The Role of the World Health Organization (WHO)

The World Health Organization began with its constitution on 7 April, 1948, a date now celebrated as World Health Day. The goal of the organization is to build a better healthier future for people all over the world. It does this through the work of more than 7000 people in over 150 countries, with six regional offices, and through its headquarters in

Geneva. WHO staff work alongside governments and other partners to ensure the highest level of health for all people. However, achievement of health goals across WHO's member states will depend on government sign-up to WHO goals, commitment and deployment of resources for health.

WHO strives to combat diseases, for example, infectious diseases such as influenza and human immunodeficiency virus (HIV), along with non-communicable disease such as heart disease and cancer. WHO also concentrates on the health of mothers and children, on the safety of breathable air, on food, on clean water and on medicines and vaccines (WHO, 2017).

Given the scale of the undertaking, it is not surprising WHO has been the subject of criticism, not least for its focus on disease prevention and eradication, whereby success in these areas is argued as elusive due to the organization being too bureaucratic and centralised to effectively and efficiently target funds and efforts (Lewis, 2003). In addition, WHO has been criticised for purported inefficiency, which prompted its director-general's to pledge renewed efforts to ensure efficiency and effectiveness are top priorities. Of greater concern though, is the criticism of WHO's focus on public health. Public health proceeds from the assumption that society as a whole should attempt to boost the health of its population through accessible healthcare, healthy environments and good individual and collective lifestyle choices. To this end WHO's commitment to public health is enshrined in its constitution, which recognises that health is not merely the absence of disease or infirmity but also a state of complete physical, mental and social well-being. This broad definition is argued by some as totalitarian, thus encouraging WHO to undertake activities in areas where it has no business (Lewis, 2003). However, the veracity of these criticisms is open to question and dependent on the perspective taken on WHO activities. For example, the WHO Framework Convention on Tobacco Control attempted to restrict tobacco advertising, sponsorship and promotion, and to establish indoor clean air controls, which critics argue infringes personal liberty and choice. People have a right to engage in risky behaviours should they wish to, or so the argument goes.

In more recent times, the World Health Organization has been severely criticised for its handling of the Ebola outbreak in West Africa in 2014. Over time and based on a number of eradication initiatives, the organization developed a standard approach to managing disease outbreaks, characterised by collating epidemic intelligence and issuing policy advice. However, following prominent failure of the malaria eradication programme, WHO's secretariat refrained from instructing governments on the precise measures they should take to eradicate or control diseases. Instead, the WHO secretariat adopted a policy of offering advice from expert consensus, and coordinating efforts only where it was explicitly invited to do so, a response which typified the approach taken throughout the latter part of the twentieth century (Kamradt-Scott, 2016). Whether or not this impacted WHO's responsibilities or whether international organizations' initial response to the Ebola crisis was appropriate and reasonable is open to debate (for a detailed discussion of the WHO's response to the 2014 Ebola outbreak in West Africa see Kamradt-Scott, 2016).

Global Health

Life expectancy is the average number of years a person has before death; conveniently calculated from birth, but may be calculated from any specified age. Dramatic improvements in life expectancy have been seen around the world throughout the twentieth century, although huge disparities exist between the richest and poorest countries. In the UK, a newborn baby boy could expect to live 79.1 years, while a newborn baby girl could expect to live 82.8 years, assuming mortality rates remain the same as they were in the UK in 2012–2014 (ons.gov.uk, 2016). Life expectancy at age 65 in the UK reached 18.4 years for men and 20.9 years for women, which means a man aged 65 could expect to live to age 83 and a woman to age 86. At age 85 a man may expect to live another 5.8 years, that is, to age 91, with a woman expecting to live for 6.8 years, that is, to nearly 92. These figures represent an increase in life expectancy over a 32-year period equivalent of an additional 3.1 months for men and 2.3 months for women. Women can still expect to live longer than men, but this gap in life expectancy at birth is narrowing over time. Life expectancy figures have obvious implications for healthcare and healthcare services in the UK. While the increase in life expectancy is considered one of the greatest achievements of the twentieth century (Britnell, 2015), nevertheless the demand this increase in life expectancy, particular in older age, places on healthcare services increases exponentially. It is self-evident that people in older age are more likely to suffer chronic disease, more likely to adopt sedentary lifestyles, and may be more likely to adopt unhealthy food choices (Bratanova, Loughnan, Klein, & Wood, 2016).

Life expectancy across the globe has increased by 5 years since 2000, the fastest rise in lifespan since the 1960s (WHO, 2016). Babies born in 2015 can expect to live to 71.4 years (73.8 years for females; 69.1 years for males). The longest lifespans are in Japan, where in 2015 newborns were expected to live to almost 84 years, followed by Switzerland, Singapore, Australia and Spain (WHO, 2016a). Life expectancy data is available by country via the Global Health Observatory Data Repository.

The degree to which older persons are susceptible in old age is subject to huge variation, dependent on important social and psychological factors and associated with poverty and wealth inequality (Bratanova et al., 2016). Nevertheless, in general terms the demand on available health resources has led the UK government to define health services as commodities while at the same time attempting to maintain an ideological commitment to universal healthcare, free at the point of delivery and available on demand. It is this mismatch between rhetoric and reality that has led to a health service in serious financial difficulty, unrest between healthcare personnel, particularly junior doctors and the Secretary of State for Health, and a deepening crisis for the NHS.

The increase in life expectancy in the UK is reflected across all nations with people everywhere living longer (WHO, 2014). Reasons for increased global life expectancy reflect a broad set of changes including a decline from high to low fertility, a steady increase in life expectancy at birth and older ages and a shift in the leading causes of death and illness from infectious and parasitic diseases to non-communicable diseases and chronic conditions. Nevertheless, the rich-poor divide persists with people in high-income countries having a much better chance of living longer than people in low-income countries. Fewer children are dying before their fifth birthday. However, it is still the case that in high-income countries a boy born in 2012 could expect to live to the age of 76; this is 16 years longer than a boy born in a low-income country, where average life expectancy is 60. For girls, the gap is even wider with a gap of 19 years separating life expectancy in high-income countries (82 years) and low-income countries (63 years). Wherever they live in the world, women can expect to live longer than men, with the greatest life expectancy for women being found in Japan, where women can expect to live to around 87 years (Ham, Dixon, & Brooke, 2012).

The gain in life expectancy in high-income countries is said to relate to success in tackling non-communicable diseases (WHO, 2014). Fewer men and women die before aged 60 years from heart disease and stroke. Richer countries are thought to have become better at managing high blood pressure, which is a significant factor in combatting cardiac and circulatory disease. On the other hand, in many sub-Saharan countries, for example, Angola, Central African Republic, Chad, Côte d'Ivoire, Democratic Republic of Congo, Lesotho, Mozambique, Nigeria and Sierra Leone, life expectancy for women and men is still less than 55 years. The number of people entering older ages will challenge national infrastructures, particularly health systems. Advancing age brings with it an increased risk of dementia, particularly Alzheimer's disease. The risk of dementia increases sharply with age, thus placing growing demands on health and long-term care as the world's population ages. Once again, this healthcare challenge, while affecting populations globally, impacts the less developed world to a far greater extent, in that low-income countries have far less resources than high-income countries to cope with the financial and social impact of the disease.

Living longer does not necessarily imply living healthier. Rises in obesity, hypertension and its associated conditions, for example, diabetes and cancer, suggest an expansion of morbidity in older age, that is, an increase in the prevalence of disability as life expectancy increases. On the other hand, changes in the rates of disability have been interpreted as indicating compression of morbidity, in other words a decrease in the prevalence of disability as life expectancy increases (NIA, NIH, 2011). Advances in medicine are also thought to impact whether or not longer lives are lived free of disability. While it is likely that technological developments in medicine will impact progression from chronic disease to disability with the result that severe disability will lessen, it is possible that milder chronic disease will increase. The high cost of managing older people with disabilities and chronic disease is generally felt most acutely in under resourced countries. However, it is also important to note that health differences exist not only between countries but between populations within countries. In general, people in higher socioeconomic circumstances experience better health across life expectancy.

Population ageing, increasing rates of dementia and increasing levels of mild, moderate and severe disability will influence how governments around the world determine health spending. However, there will continue to be vast differences between developed and developing countries in terms of available resources for healthcare. In developed countries, acute and long-term care are widely available, whereas in developing countries acute and institutional long-term care are less well developed. While little is currently known about the impact of ageing populations and associated healthcare costs on the developing world (NIA, NIH, 2011), nevertheless the cost of an ageing population is likely to be felt more acutely in low-income countries.

Global Standards for Nurse Education

There are an estimated 35 million nurses and midwives, making up the greater part of the global healthcare workforce (WHO, 2009). While nurses and midwives across the globe contribute in all areas of healthcare delivery from primary care to acute and long-term care in community settings, their contribution to policy making around healthcare and to high-level decision-making on health issues is often limited. The degree to which nurses and midwives are involved in shaping healthcare policy and organization is thought to reflect the status of nurses and midwives and the general level of education of the profession in a given country. The contribution that nurses and midwives can make to the health of nations was recognised in 2001 by the World Health Assembly (WHA). Resolution WHA54.12 validated the World Health Organization's (WHO) commitment to scaling up the health professions and established a number of imperatives: (a) for member States to give urgent attention to ways of improving nursing and midwifery in their respective countries and (b) for the Director General to prepare an action plan, with inbuilt evaluation procedures for strengthening nursing and midwifery services (The Strategic Directions for Strengthening Nursing and Midwifery Services 2002–2004). A further resolution (WHA59.23) supported the development of global standards for initial nursing and midwifery education as key to strengthening nursing and midwifery services and meeting Millennium Development Goals for Health. The need for global standards had arisen due to increasing complexities in healthcare provision, increasing numbers of health professionals at different levels and the need to assure more equitable access to healthcare. In recognising complexities in healthcare provision and inequities in the quality of nursing and midwifery education globally, the World Health Organization officially made the link between standards of initial nursing and midwifery education and the quality of the nursing and midwifery workforce and in so doing paved the way for the establishment of global standards for the initial education of professional nurses and midwives, subsequently published in 2009.

The goal of the global standards for initial nursing and midwifery education was to establish educational criteria and assure outcomes that are based on evidence and competency, to promote progressive education and lifelong learning, to ensure employment of practitioners competent to provide quality care and to promote positive health outcomes in the populations they serve (WHO, 2009). Key to achievement of these goals was the need to establish all initial education at university level. However, while university programmes are well established in some member countries, other countries have different levels and systems for nursing and midwifery education.

The global standards require initial programmes to ensure graduates are able to demonstrate competencies in nursing and midwifery practice and demonstrate understanding of the determinants of health and can meet local regulatory body requirements. However, no mention is made of the implications of this requirement for member countries where regulation is either absent or poorly developed. The standards require graduates of initial nursing and midwifery programmes should be able to use evidence to underpin practice and should be culturally competent and able to practise in the healthcare systems of their respective countries and meet population needs. In addition, programme graduates should be critical thinkers, able to manage resources and to practise safely and effectively and have leadership ability, community orientation and the ability to act as client advocate and to work with professional partners. The World Health Organization, in setting these standards, recognised particular issues may limit immediate implementation of the global standards including the requirement for all initial programmes to be at university level. In so doing WHO recognised the standards as aspirational for many member countries rather than achievable, at least in the short term.

In terms of curriculum design, the global standards require schools of nursing and midwifery to design curricula to deliver programmes that take account of workforce planning and national and international healthcare polices. Classroom and clinical learning should be a feature of initial programmes, although no reference is made to the ratio of theory to practice, save for the need for programmes to balance theoretical and practice components of the curriculum. Mention is made of the need to use recognised approaches to learning and teaching in programmes including, but not limited to adult education, self-directed learning, e-learning and clinical simulation (WHO, 2009, p. 24). Notable by its absence is any mention of critical pedagogy in nursing and midwifery education despite the reference to the need for graduates to develop critical and analytical thinking, community service orientation, leadership and continual professional development. Critical pedagogy has the power to shift how students think about the issues affecting their lives and the world at large, potentially energising them to seize such moments as possibilities for acting on the world and for engaging it as a matter of politics, power and social justice (Giroux, 2006, p. 66). Given the World Health Organization comment that of the 35 million nurses and midwives making up the greater part of the global healthcare workforce very few are in a position to impact strategic decisions around health strategy and policy, the absence of critical pedagogy is counterintuitive to espoused goals for initial nurse education.

Global Standards for Nurse Educators

The World Health Organization followed its work on global standards for nursing and midwifery education with work to develop core competencies for nurse educators. In so doing WHO recognised the preparation of nurse educators is critical to the development of knowledge, skills and attitudes of nurses. In making the argument that a competent workforce is central to achieving universal health coverage (WHO, 2006), an imperative is created not just for a competency-based approach to the initial preparation of nurses but for a competency-based approach to curricula for nurse educator programmes. A four-step process followed, beginning with a comprehensive literature review on the subject of nurse educator competency, including global policy documents, literature from professional health councils and associations and research articles examining the competence and preparation of the health practitioner faculty (WHO, 2016). The review resulted in formulation of 28 Nurse Educator Core Competencies. Step two in the process involved a Global Delphi Survey to garner expert input on the essential competences required of nurse educators. The original 28 core competency statements were converted into a survey format subsequently sent to 20 nurse educators, of whom 13 responded. These original competency statements were then revised following survey feedback, resulting in a total of 49 core competencies for nurse educators, organised within 13 domains. A second survey followed, whereby 71 participants from worldwide nursing organizations, ostensibly representing the global nursing and midwifery professions, were asked to respond to all 49 competency statements. Quantitative survey data combined with qualitative comments provided the basis for a competency framework, which was then subjected to step three; the validation process.

Validation of the Nurse Educator Core Competencies (NECC) involved a number of stages involving consultation at various levels. A final review culminated in 8 broad competency domains and 37 core competencies. A fourth and final step in the development process saw further categorisation of competencies within cognitive (knowledge), affective (attitudes and behaviours) and psychomotor (skill) domains.

While cognitive, affective and psychomotor learning domains are identified across eight competency domains, the World Health Organization believe nurse educators will merge knowledge, skills and behaviours in any given situation towards optimum or ideal performance. Such performance complexity, they suggest, calls for integration of teaching and learning domains to reduce repetitious and redundant elements in the design of curricula (WHO, 2016a, p. 10).

In framing core competencies for nurse educators within cognitive, affective and psychomotor domains, the World Health Organization implicitly draw on a framework not dissimilar to Bloom's Taxonomy of Educational Objectives (Bloom, Englehart, Furst, Hill, & Krathwohl, 1956). Developed by a committee of college and university examiners between 1949 and 1954 the taxonomy provides a classification of the goals of the educational process, whereby educational objectives are organised within cognitive, affective and psychomotor domains. Bloom et al.'s taxonomy is premised on the belief that the higher-order skills of analysis, synthesis and evaluation are essential to education at all levels.

Acquisition of these higher-order skills necessarily requires critical thinking skills on the part of teachers, in as much as learning to think critically is to learn how to ask and answer questions of analysis, synthesis and evaluation. Taxonomies such as this, organise cognitive processes into a one-way hierarchy, premised on the idea that knowledge is always a simpler behaviour than comprehension, comprehension a simpler behaviour than application, application a simpler behaviour than analysis and analysis a simpler behaviour than synthesis and evaluation. This is misleading in that achieving knowledge always presupposes at least a minimal level of comprehension, in this case a minimal understanding of critical thinking.

The global standards for nurse educators presuppose a minimal understanding of critical thinking as a prerequisite for achievement of higher-order skills (analysis, synthesis, evaluation). However, in the absence of critical thinking skills, the achievement of higher-order skills is compromised, thus making it unlikely for critical thinking and higher-order skills to transfer from teacher to learner.

In as much as the World Health Organization has made efforts to address the quality of nursing services and of nurse education worldwide through its work around global standards, as a means to address global health needs, nevertheless the perverse effect has seen an increase in migration of the nursing and midwifery workforce.

A Migratory Nursing Workforce

Throughout the world, the supply of skilled nurses and midwives is notoriously volatile, with major shifts into and out of the workforce as economies fluctuate (Pittman, 2013). Nursing shortages in developed countries accelerates international nursing recruitment and migration, leading to debate about the consequences for sending and receiving countries and for the meeting of global health needs (Aiken, Buchan, Sochalski, Nichols, & Powell, 2004). While well-educated nurses are able to migrate to countries offering better working conditions, this phenomenon invariably affects low-income countries to a greater degree than higher income countries (low-income countries are defined in July each year by the world bank, e.g. in 2015, as countries with a gross national income per capita [GNI] of $1025, www.worldbank.org). The escalating requirements for nurses in developed countries depletes the supply of qualified nurses in less developed countries, for example, the Philippines, whereby its government-approved programme has produced nurses for export. While international recruitment of nurses is not a new phenomenon, recruitment from developing countries exacerbates the shortage of nurses, impacts quality of nursing care and mitigates the opportunity for developing countries to meet WHO millennium goals.

While it may be expedient for developing countries to adopt global standards for nursing programmes and global standards for nurse educator programmes, nevertheless this may lead to an increase in nursing migration at least in the short term. Once qualified to a global standard, overseas nurses are an attractive proposition for developed countries. The depletion of supply of qualified nurses in less developed countries thus cripples their healthcare systems. As a result, low-income countries benefit less from the World Health Organization's aspirations to address complexities in healthcare provision than developed countries. In the UK, the Nursing and Midwifery Council, in a controversial move, has rescinded the requirement for overseas nurses to complete 3 months of supervised practice, as the NHS attempts solutions to its staffing crisis. The NMC insists that the approach to overseas registration is an internationally recognised and rigorous way of ensuring that those applying for registration who trained overseas are able to practise safely and effectively in the UK. While the implications of this move are yet to be seen, the policy is certain to impact countries whose nursing workforce is drained in order to bolster the nursing workforce of more affluent countries.

Nurses migrate to the UK and to other countries for a variety of personal, social and financial reasons. Some countries, despite domestic healthcare needs, are not able to create enough jobs for the health professionals they train, which serves to increase motivations to emigrate. Poor wages, economic instability and poorly resourced healthcare systems 'push' nurses to leave developing countries, while at the same time better working and living conditions 'pull' nurses towards developed countries. While the push and pull factors exert a strong effect on nursing migration, the reality often does not live up to expectation. Allan and Larsen (2003) in an extensive report commissioned by the RCN reported on the experiences of internationally recruited nurses working in the UK. International nurses working in different sectors and geographical regions of the UK provided insight into the reality of migration including poor accommodation and lack of personal support. International nurses reported not being able to use their nursing qualifications and being prevented from using the nursing skills they had practised in their home countries. International nurses reported feeling under-valued and, in some cases, being subject to discrimination and worse still to 'crude racism' (Allan & Larsen, 2003, p. 4). While much work has been done since this report by the NHS to address the poor experiences of international nurses, nevertheless the impact on the lives of nurses from both sending and receiving countries extends beyond the policy decision to address nursing workforce issues through international recruitment. The continued demand for overseas nurses requires ethical recruitment guidelines, which not only consider the needs of developing countries from which nurses are drawn, but always takes account of the working conditions of the receiving countries, especially as they are experienced by the migratory nursing workforce.

The NHS is currently facing a major shortfall in nurses, exacerbated by the result of the EU referendum in 2016. A report from the Institute for Employment Studies revealed around 4.5% of nurses working in the NHS in the year before the referendum had come from EU countries (excluding Ireland), which showed a steep increase from 2009 where it was reported to be 1%. Some reassurance has been given that nurses who have been working in the NHS for 5 years will have the right to remain; however, it is not clear what the situation will be for those who do not meet this criterion. While health ministers have repeatedly called on the government for clarification, no such guarantee has been forthcoming, at least not until reciprocal arrangements have been agreed as part of the ongoing negotiations between Britain and the European Union (EU). One partial solution might be to name nursing as a protected profession. However, the difficulties therein lie in devising a set of criteria, which allow nurses to remain, or come to Britain when other occupations with similar shortages are not afforded the same consideration. An alternative solution might be to increase nursing recruitment from countries outside the EU. However, this is difficult to do with respect to government controls over immigration. More to the point though is the moral and ethical arguments against such a policy as the shortage of nurses is a global phenomenon, so much so that one country's policy to address the shortfalls affects another, whether directly or indirectly.

Conclusion

This chapter has considered ways in which global health services and subsequent nurse education has developed to meet local needs. The chapter has argued that increasing longevity coupled with exponential increases in long-term, complex health conditions is a global phenomenon, causing governments worldwide to rethink how healthcare is conceptualised and subsequently funded. Low-income countries and low-income families within countries suffer most in terms of access to healthcare, thus suffering poorer health outcomes than their wealthier counterparts. Continued commitment to universal healthcare in the UK, free at the point of delivery and available to all, has seen the NHS in recent times experience its worst financial difficulties since inception in 1948.

The World Health Organization, through development of global standards for initial nurse education, coupled with global standards for nurse educator programmes has attempted to address increasing complexities in health and increasing numbers of health professionals at different levels. However, the perverse effect is a better educated workforce and thus able to migrate from lower income countries where work opportunities are limited to high-income countries where working conditions are more favourable. The UK government is complicit in this in permitting the NMC to relax its requirement for overseas nurses to undertake periods of supervised practice before being allowed to practise. The experiences of internationally recruited nurses to the UK have been shown to be compromised in terms of poor support, poor use of skills and in some cases reported racism.

The following chapter argues for a rethinking of nurse education to incorporate critical pedagogy as a means of preparing students for contemporary nursing work.

References

Aiken, L. H., Buchan, J., Sochalski, J., Nichols, B., & Powell, M. (2004). Trends in international nurse migration. *Health Affairs, 23*(3), 69–77.

Allan, H. T., & Larsen, J. A. (2003). *"We need respect": Experiences of internationally recruited nurses in the UK*. London: RCN.

Bloom, B., Englehart, M., Furst, E., Hill, W., & Krathwohl, D. (1956). *Taxonomy of educational objectives: The classification of educational goals. Handbook I: Cognitive domain*. New York, Toronto: Longmans, Green.

Bratanova, B., Loughnan, S., Klein, O., & Wood, R. (2016). The rich get richer, the poor get even: Perceived socio-economic position influences micro-social distribution of wealth. *Scandinavian Journal of Psychology, 57*(3), 243–249.

Britnell, M. (2015). *In search of the perfect health system*. London: Palgrave Macmillan.

Giroux, H. A. (2006). Higher education under siege: Implications for public intellectuals. *The NEA Higher Education Journal*, Fall, 63–78.

Ham, C., Dixon, A., & Brooke, B. (2012). *Transforming the delivery of health and social care: The case for fundamental change*. London: The King's Fund.

Kamradt-Scott, A. (2016). WHO's to blame? The World Health Organization and the 2014 Ebola outbreak in West Africa. *Third World Quarterly, 37*(3), 401–418, published online: 4 Jan 2016.

Lewis, N. (2003). World health organization profile: Criticisms of WHO. Retrieved April 26, 2017, from http://health.howstuffworks.com/medicine/health/care/who5.htm

NIH National Institute on Aging. (2011). Longer lives and disability. Retrieved from https://auth.nia.nih.gov/research/publication/global-health-and-aging/longer-lives-and-disability

Office for National Statistics (ONS). (2016). Office for National Statistics (ONS), [GB]. Retrieved from https://www.ons.gov.uk/peoplepopulationandcommunity/birthsdeathsandmarriages/lifeexpectancies/bulletins/pastandprojecteddatafromtheperiodandcohortlifetables/2014baseduk1981to2064#life-expectancy-ex-at-birth-in-the-uk

Pittman, P. (2013). Nursing workforce education, migration and the quality of health care: A global challenge. *International Journal for Quality in Health Care, 25*(4), 349–351.

Shah, A. (2011). Health care around the world. Retrieved from http://www.globalissues.org/article/774/health-care-around-the-world#TheUSandHealthCare

WHO. (2006). *Working together for health*. The World Health Report. The World Health Organisation, Geneva.

WHO. (2009). *Global standards for the initial education of professional nurses and midwives*. Geneva: World Health Organisation.

WHO. (2014). *World health statistics 2014*. Geneva: World Health Organisation.

WHO. (2016). *Global Health Observatory data. World Health Statistics 2016: Monitoring health for the SDGs*. Retrieved December 14, 2016, from www.who.int/gho/publications/world_health_statistics/2016/en/

WHO. (2017). About WHO: Who we are, what we do. Retrieved from http://www.who.int/about/en/

4

Pedagogy in Nurse Education

Nurse education in the UK is delivered within a tightly regulated framework, wherein programmes are required to conform to a set of prescribed standards and outcome measures. In the wake of the initial Francis Inquiry in 2010, the NMC revisited and published new standards for pre-registration nursing education, which placed significant emphasis on care and compassion for patients (NMC, 2013). Nurse educators design nursing curricula to prepare students to challenge and critique nursing practice within this 'conventional pedagogical' framework, which determines what nurses need to know and how nursing knowledge and skills are verified in both the theory and practice setting. Conventional pedagogy such as this is characterised by the need to transmit those skills, facts and standards of moral and social conduct considered necessary, and is imposed from above and outside (Dewey, 1938). Nurse teachers are the instrument by which nursing knowledge is conveyed and behaviours consistent with nursing are enforced. In this sense, conventional nurse education is imposed from above.

Conventional pedagogy proliferates in nurse education for reasons that, without standards and verifiable outcome measures, the NMC would have difficulty in meeting its public obligation to ensure that nurses and midwives provide high-quality standards of care to their patients and clients (NMC, 2010). As such, the NMC is rightly concerned to 'publicly' address the concerns that nurses are failing to deliver care with compassion. The tension for nurse educators, is to design nursing curricula to prepare students to challenge and critique nursing practice, within the confines of a pedagogical framework where the object is to assure the public of the knowledge, skills and good character of all nurses (and midwives) admitted to the register (NMC, 2015b).

Critical pedagogy, in contrast, is bottom-up, or characterised by teaching which attempts to help students question and challenge domination, and the beliefs and practices that dominate them (Freire, 1972). Critical pedagogy is not a prescriptive set of practices—it is a continuous moral project (Coles, 2014). In this sense, critical pedagogy is eminently suited to nurse education, as it strives to prepare student nurses for the challenge of nursing practice.

This chapter argues for a rethinking of nurse education to incorporate critical pedagogy, as a means of preparing students for contemporary nursing work. The work of Paulo Freire and Henry Giroux is considered of particular relevance for nurse education, as both offer insight into ways of thinking about present-day, modern nursing, which takes account of the social, political and technological context of healthcare. Jack Mezirow's work on adult learning provides a critical lens through which to view the role of the nursing curriculum in the development of sustainable positive nursing practice.

The argument made in this book thus far is that regulation of nurse education in response to criticisms of nursing practice and nurse education has resulted in positivist approaches to design and delivery of nursing curricula. Nurse educators struggle to act with agency to develop appropriate pedagogies within the confines of a tightly regulated and constricted framework. Pedagogical strategies for nurse education are key to delivering aspirations for nurse education. However, conventional approaches to nursing pedagogy have predominated over time, with nurse educators constrained by the canons of educational institutions and the regulatory body. Critical pedagogy, underpinned by critical theory, attends to situations where social agency is denied (McLean, 2008).

For this reason, an exploration of the potential for critical pedagogy as a transformative agent in nurse education is both relevant and timely. First though, in order to provide context for consideration of critical pedagogy in contemporary nurse education it is important to understand something of its history.

Historical Developments Shaping Nurse Education

Nurse education in the UK has seen an intense transformation over the last 25 years, from a largely apprenticeship model of 'training' with heavy emphasis on the acquisition of clinical skills to a more educative model, with emphasis on knowledge acquisition alongside clinical competency. Apprenticeship models tended to be framed within a largely biomedical, behaviourally focused, positivist paradigm where the objective was to train nurses to become members of a community of nurses, historically subservient to the medical profession. Over time the traditional approach to training nurses, at first almost exclusively located in clinical settings, has given way to education located in schools of nursing, followed by colleges of nursing, and since the early 1990s, within universities.

The changes to ways in which nurses are taught the art and science of nursing are a response to a number of key reports, the most influential being the Report of the Committee of Nursing (1972). The Committee, set up in June 1970 under the Chairmanship of Professor Asa Briggs was charged with reviewing the role of the nurse and midwife in the hospital and the community and the education and training required for that role, so that the best use is made of available manpower to meet present needs and the needs of an integrated health service. The Briggs Committee, as it became known, considered a new educational and training structure to be of key importance in producing nurses for a caring profession. The structure proposed by the Briggs Committee included two grades of nurses, one certified, one registered, in which early training was to be identical, leading to a Certificate of Nursing Practice, common to all branches of nursing including midwifery. Students wishing to study further were able to continue, with further training leading to registration.

After some 6 years of debate and delay regarding the recommendations of the Briggs Committee, the Nurses, Midwives and Health Visitors Act (1979) was passed and a number of changes were made to regulatory structures, including the establishment of a unified central council: the United Kingdom Central Council for Nursing, Midwifery and Health Visiting (UKCC), whose remit included responsibility for professional standards, education and discipline. The UKCC was replaced in 2002 by the Nursing and Midwifery Council (NMC), who subsequently took over the quality functions previously under the remit of the English National Board (ENB) (Eaton, 2012). The Briggs Report paved the way for the later changes to pre-registration nursing, which ultimately resulted in Project 2000 (Peate, 2013).

Project 2000 saw a transfer of nurse education from a 'training' model based largely in hospital settings to an 'education' model based in academic settings, usually universities. The academic level was established at a minimum of a higher education diploma. Further changes to the standards of pre-registration nursing education programmes by the NMC have seen all programmes now delivered at undergraduate level within the university setting, with successful candidates exiting entry-level nursing programmes with a first degree and eligibility for entry onto the NMC register.

In spite of developments, in terms of structure, location, entry and exit levels within initial nursing programmes since the Report of the Committee of Nursing in 1972, thinking around appropriate pedagogy for nursing has not been well considered. While nurses are well educated in terms of theory to underpin practice, nevertheless and in terms of nursing praxis (theory in action), contemporary nursing practice requires more of nurses than the ability to practise competently. Contemporary nursing practice requires nurses who are critically aware, who can engage in client advocacy, and who are capable of socially conscious practice. While the vision and mission of most nursing programmes recognises the need to go beyond preparing nurses for the workplace, a largely restrictive, proscribed curriculum restricts the capacity for nurse education to fully prepare nurses to work and to live well in present-day, modern nursing.

Nurses have a right to expect nurse education should equip them with knowledge and skills to enable them to recognise, examine and address the flaws in the contemporary nursing workplace. Nurse educators have a responsibility to carefully determine pedagogy, and to design nursing curricula to enable students to not only practise competently but to know the important distinction between what is 'good enough' and what should not, should never, be tolerated. Critical pedagogy for nurse education is the means by which nurses are educated not only to know this difference, but also to have the skills to act when care is unacceptable and be assured that concerns about care, raised in good faith, will be robustly addressed.

Pedagogy in nurse education is concerned with what nurses need to know in order to understand nursing as a social enterprise, as a political activity, as a technically demanding profession, in a digital age, and where patients, families and carers have access to medical and health-related information on a global scale. The goal of nurse education is thus to prepare nurses to meet the challenges of contemporary nursing practice. However, despite this rhetoric, pedagogy in nurse education has not kept pace with societal, organisational and technological change. Instead nurse education continues to display elements of apprenticeship style training reminiscent of nurse training prior to the introduction of Project 2000.

Conventional Pedagogy in Nurse Education

Apprenticeship style training in nurse education relies on occupational expertise and identity, social and personal maturity, and locational or close association between the qualified nurse and the student. Apprenticeship models, whereby novitiates learn from experts through induction into a community of practice work well in situations of relative stability (Lave & Wenger, 1991). However, when ideal conditions for apprenticeship cannot be met, for example, poor staffing levels and over-reliance on agency and international nursing staff who are themselves navigating new and unfamiliar learning environments, the learning environment is compromised learning such that learners find themselves having to 'sink or swim' (Hughes & Fraser, 2011). Despite the best efforts of nurse educators and practitioners to 'bridge' the theory practice gap by recourse to strategies such as mentorship, continuous assessment of practice, reflective assignments and other collaborative learning and teaching strategies, these attempts are thwarted by environments which are not conducive to and cannot effectively support the learner (O'Kane, 2012).

The concerns around apprenticeship models of training are by no means held by all, with high-profile figures implicitly advocating a return to apprenticeship style training. In the wake of the Francis Inquiry into Mid Staffordshire NHS Foundation Trust, Camilla Cavendish was asked by the Secretary of State for Health to review what could be done to ensure that unregistered staff in the National Health Service (NHS) and social care treat all patients and clients with care and compassion. Cavendish concluded that systems which care for the public are disconnected. The NHS, she says, operates in silos, and social care is seen as a distant land occupied by a different tribe (The Cavendish Review, 2013, p. 5). The Cavendish Review, as an antidote to this disconnected landscape recommends significant changes to recruitment, training and education, in particular that the NMC should make caring experiences a prerequisite to starting a nursing degree. However, the Review does not comment on how the disconnected landscape of health and social care might support potential nursing students to develop 'attitudes and aptitudes for caring' (p. 9). Since publication of the Cavendish Review the government has announced a new scheme to develop a nursing apprenticeship standard. The 'trailblazer group', as it is known, under the direction of the Department for Business, Innovation and Skills are developing a degree level apprenticeship which will widen access to nursing. The new apprenticeship will make sure there is an opportunity for talented care workers to progress into nursing, giving them a route to advance their careers and a chance to use their vocational experience of working as a healthcare assistant to enter the nursing profession. Furthermore, the trailblazer group will look at how to ensure that on completion, apprentices will have all the skills, knowledge and confidence they need to perform nursing duties well and confidently, meeting their employer's and professional registration requirements (Gov.UK, 2014).

The government response to the Cavendish Review, which in turn was a government response to the Francis Inquiry, is clearly to focus attention away from the central findings of the Francis Inquiry of institutional failings at every level, in favour of a focus on recruitment, training and education of nurses. In so doing, the government implicitly shifted the responsibility for the reported lack of care and compassion at Mid Staffs Foundation Hospital Trust to the nursing workforce (qualified and support staff), rather than addressing the serious concerns identified by the Francis Inquiry, around organisational and structural issues within the health service, including management and leadership at every level (Francis Report, 2013).

Conventional Pedagogy and the Theory-Practice Gap in Nursing

Conventional pedagogy in nurse education is predicated on the integration of theory and practice, with equal emphasis placed on theoretical knowledge to underpin practice and acquisition of practical nursing competencies. Nursing programmes assess both practical and theoretical elements, though often in different ways, for example, written assignments to assess knowledge and continuous assessment of practice to assess clinical competency. Formal separation between clinical learning and classroom learning is thought to impede the ability of nurses to integrate knowledge, technical skills and ethical practice.

Continuous situated 'coaching' is posited as an antidote to the theory-practice gap, in that the method allows students to understand all the factors in specific situations that are subject to change; the importance of signs and symptoms; the patients, families and other healthcare workers' requests; the available resources; and any constraints present (Pagnucci, Carnevale, Bagnasco, & Sasso, 2015). However, situated coaching is predicated on the assumption that immersion in clinical situations, which are subject to change, predisposes nursing students to be able to make decisions in unpredictable and continuously changing circumstances, in other words enables the transference of learning from one situation to another. While situated coaching may bring benefits in terms of integration of theory and practice through exposure to rapidly changing situations, this can by no means be guaranteed. The high level of attrition currently experienced from undergraduate nursing programmes, reported to be in part associated with the stress incurred through clinical placements, is suggestive that often the clinical environment is not conducive to learning. Fear of making mistakes around clinical procedures, conflict between the ideal and real practice on the wards, unfriendly atmosphere and being reprimanded in front of staff and patients are all cited as reasons why nursing students leave the profession (Orton, 2011). Pedagogical strategies, which by their very nature place students under continuous stress, should be underpinned by robust evidence of effectiveness in the cultivation of learning.

Pedagogy in nursing should be concerned with the nature of knowledge and learning, including how knowledge is produced, negotiated, transformed and realised in the interaction between the teacher, the student and the knowledge itself (Ironside, 2001). Conventional pedagogy assumes that learning is rational, orderly and a sequential process that leads to cognitive gain and the acquisition of specific skills. Conventional pedagogy is predominantly teacher-centred, with the teacher's knowledge being privileged and superior to both the student's knowledge and experience, despite the fact that a student's experience of healthcare may be more recent than that of the teacher.

Conventional pedagogies are characterised by teaching is telling, knowledge is facts, and learning is recall. Students are treated as spectators in the learning process who are focused on solutions and answers already known; theory is presented out of context or within limited contexts with the learner subordinated to the teacher. The problem with conventional pedagogy in nursing lies in its inability to develop critical thinking skills essential for contemporary nursing practice. An antidote to the deficiencies of conventional approaches to nurse education may be found by recourse to critical pedagogy.

Critical Pedagogy and Its Importance to Nurse Education: The Work of Paulo Freire and Henry Giroux

Critical pedagogy has evolved over many decades. However, it remains as relevant today as in the 1960s and 1970s, where it developed as a reaction among academics to the repeated failure of socialist governments around the world to deliver promises of economic equality (Hicks, 2004). The goal of critical pedagogy is to challenge conservative, right wing and traditional philosophies and politics. For this reason, critical pedagogy is essential to contemporary nursing practice, in that nurses, while constituting the largest part of the health sector workforce historically, struggle to contribute fully to policy-making around healthcare and to high-level decision-making on health issues (WHO, 2009).

Critical pedagogy draws on critical theory, which relates to an ideal standard or mode of being, grounded in justice and freedom. 'Critical' within nurse education refers to a critique both of the conditions in which nurse education operates and to a critique of nurse educators' knowledge and understanding of these conditions. Critique involves reflection on what has been taken for granted, identifying constraints to injustice and freeing oneself to consider fairer alternatives. Critical theory raises consciousness, empowering the critical educator to challenge the 'taken for granted' while allowing for structural constraints to be acknowledged. Critical theory supports the critical educator to question the hidden assumptions and purposes of existing forms of practice.

Proponents of critical theory advocate that individuals are essentially unfree and inhabit a world rife with contradictions and asymmetries of power and privilege (McLaren, 2009). It follows that critical educators endorse theories, which are dialectical, that is, which recognise the problems of society as more than isolated events of individuals or deficiencies in social structure. Problems are seen as forming part of the interactive context between individual and society with the individual and society inextricably interwoven. Dialectical critical theory involves searching out apparent contradictions, for example, the contradictory role of the NMC, who on the one hand devolve responsibility for design and administration of nursing programmes to higher education institutions and on the other hand prescribe educational standards, which nursing programmes must adhere to. Dialectical critical theory requires the critical educator to engage in thinking which reflects back and forth between elements of part and whole; to focus "simultaneously on both sides of a social contradiction" (McLaren, 2009, p. 61).

Critical pedagogy has been defined in different ways by critical theorists in a variety of disciplines (education, psychology, sociology). Of these critical theorists, the work of Paulo Freire and Henry Giroux is of particular relevance to nurse education and nursing practice, for reasons that both believe the purpose of education is not simply to reproduce conditions to maintain the status quo, but to resist, critique and transform conditions for a more just and equitable society for all.

Paulo Freire, perhaps the most celebrated writer on critical pedagogy provides much that is useful to nurse education. Freire developed a pedagogic theory for use in literacy programmes in Brazil in the 1970s, of which three central ideas are relevant to the current context for nurse education. Freire proposed the notion of critical consciousness, which allows people to question the nature of their historical and social situation and to 'read the world' with the goal of acting as subjects in the creation of a democratic society (Freire, 1985). Education for Freire implies a dialogic exchange between teachers and students, where both learn, both question, both reflect and both participate in making sense of any given situation or learning experience (Freire, 1972). This notion of critical consciousness is of immediate relevance to nurse education as it seeks to influence ways in which nursing students are prepared for the world of nursing work. Freire argued for teachers to be endowed with the central role of creating environments in which students are likely to engage in learning that is authentic. In other words, teachers need to identify with their students in order to bring about a mutual understanding of the goals of the education process. At the heart of Freire's pedagogy was an anti-authoritarian, dialogical and interactive approach, which aimed to examine issues of relational power for students and workers (McLaren, 2009). While nurse education is regulated by the NMC, and framed within a competency-based model, nevertheless nurse educators need to develop innovative and creative approaches to nurse education, which places at the heart of educational experiences analysis of the social and political context in which health services are organised and delivered, in addition to educating towards competency in practice. Freire clearly informed the thinking of Giroux, in that teaching is a profoundly moral enterprise.

Henry Giroux has been called the father of critical pedagogy, a claim he disputes when pointing out that while playing a prominent role in its development, critical pedagogy emerged out of a long series of educational struggles that extend from the work of Paulo Freire in Brazil to the work advanced by Roger Simon, David Livingstone and Joe Kincheloe in the 1970s and through into the 1980s. According to Giroux critical pedagogy signals how questions of audience, power and evaluation actively work to construct particular relations between teachers and students, institutions and society, classrooms and communities. Giroux makes a key point when suggesting that critical pedagogy is a movement, an ongoing struggle, which takes place in many different social formations and places. Contemporary nursing practice, as a social formation and place, is thus ideally placed to benefit from pedagogy which takes as its central tenet education as both a political and moral project, and not simply a technique, that is, a way of teaching specific nursing knowledge to underpin acquisition of nursing competencies. Nursing requires more than this; likewise nurse education should aspire to deliver more than this.

Pedagogy, according to Giroux, is always political because it is connected to the acquisition of agency. As a political project, pedagogy illuminates the relationships among knowledge, authority and power, drawing attention to questions concerning who has control over the conditions for the production of knowledge, values and skills (Giroux, 2011). Critical pedagogy illuminates how knowledge, identities and authority are constructed within particular sets of social relations. For Giroux, critical pedagogy is concerned with teaching students not only to think, but to come to grips with a sense of individual and social responsibility, and what it means to be responsible for one's actions as part of a broader attempt to be an engaged citizen who can expand and deepen the possibilities of democratic public life. Given nursing students are preparing for a profession where critical awareness is vitally important, it is essential for nurse education to be underpinned by pedagogical approaches which espouse a belief in democratic education and which promote a culture of concern for others, an ethic of care and a deep understanding and empathy for human suffering.

Transformation Theory and Its Importance to Nurse Education: The Work of Jack Mezirow

Healthcare in the UK is currently facing unprecedented financial and operational pressures, due in part to increasing demand for services, in particular emergency care, although demand on other services has also increased (Maguire, Dunn, & Mckenna, 2016). A changing demographic profile, whereby people are living longer with complex illness and disability has seen the cost of providing care free at the point of delivery spiralling upwards such that the NHS now faces the biggest overspend in its history (Campbell, 2016). Within this context nurses are expected to have the knowledge, skills and behaviours to be autonomous, discerning and technologically skilled practitioners. As such nurse education is pivotal in ensuring nurses are equipped with the knowledge and skills needed for the provision of high-quality care for all client groups, wherever healthcare is needed. Consequently, nurse education needs to remain responsive to the changing needs, developments, priorities and expectations in health and healthcare (NMC, 2010). The challenge for nurse educators is to develop a curriculum which educates student nurses to be competent and skilled practitioners, while at the same time places emphasis on the importance of life-long learning as the route towards sustainable positive nursing practice. Transformation theory when used to inform nursing pedagogy facilitates sustainable development of nurse education, in other words a responsive dynamic and evolving nursing curriculum, as opposed to a static, inflexible and reactive curriculum (Renigere, 2014).

Transformation theory is the cumulation of extensive grounded research undertaken by Jack Mezirow, beginning in the late twentieth century and continuing into the early twenty-first century. Through transformation theory Mezirow explains how transformative learning occurs, what that learning involves and how it is developed in the adult learner. Transformation theory implies a non-reversible shift in the learner's perspective towards greater inclusiveness, discrimination, openness or permeability (to other ideas), flexibility, reflexiveness and autonomy, which Mezirow termed a shift in the person's meaning perspective. A meaning perspective is a basic belief or assumption a person holds about how the world works (Mezirow, 1978, 1991). Important within transformation theory is the idea that transformative learning occurs when an adult engages in activities that cause or allow them to see a different worldview from their own. For the learning to be transformative, adults then work to integrate the implications of that different worldview into their own worldview, thereby enlarging it.

Mezirow, in developing the idea of a transformation of a meaning perspective drew on the work of Kuhn who described the idea of a paradigm shift. A paradigm is a set of concepts, beliefs, methods of enquiry and values that are held by a particular scientific discipline, which tend towards forms of inquiry and research that reinforce these same concepts, beliefs and values (Kuhn, 1970). A paradigm shift has been commonly used to describe a shift in the debate about a range of methodological practices in research (Denscombe, 2008). However, Mezirow applied the use of the term 'paradigm shift' to an individual as a result of a transformative learning experience. He argued that a transformative learning shift always leads an individual towards improved psychological health and as a consequence this flows onto the community generally through improved social and cultural outcomes derived from individual actions. This is seen as essential in nursing given the context in which contemporary nursing is practised. Transformative learning experiences when embodied within the nursing curriculum have potential to 'shift' the learner away from narrow, problematic, fixed or static meaning perspectives towards more inclusive, discriminating, open, flexible, holistic and flexible meaning perspectives. These perspectives are synonymous with nursing, which makes transformation theory eminently relevant to transformational pedagogy in nurse education.

The relevance of Mezirow's transformation theory to nursing is clear, in that nursing as art, science and as a moral enterprise requires nursing students, and indeed practising nurses to embrace the worldview of the other person. This is often challenging, not least because of cultural differences, or due to the learner holding a worldview inconsistent with the worldview of the 'other' person, or the one being cared for. The concept of transformation theory is fundamental to the shift in meaning perspective necessary in learning about nursing, and to the lifelong learning, which is required for the development of sustainable nursing practice. Transformation theory has potential to inform approaches to learning and teaching about nursing while at the same time paying attention to the psychological health and well-being of the learner nurse, thereby impacting attrition from nurse education programmes and contributing to a future healthy workforce.

It is important to note Mezirow's transformation theory has been criticised for its narrow focus on individual transformation (Wang & Sarbo, 2004). This is an important acknowledgement in the context of contemporary nursing practise, whereby individual practitioners are often expected to change their behaviour, as opposed to organisational behaviour change, which is usually argued to be dependent on resources and/or prohibited by cost. Despite the criticism of transformation theory, nevertheless, the theory has potential to transform the nursing curriculum when used to underpin a philosophy for nurse education and/or a framework for curriculum design. In so doing two important parallels are drawn between nurse education and how adults learn, namely, that both are context dependent and therefore require contextually adapted philosophies for learning and teaching.

Contextually Adapted Philosophies for Learning and Teaching About Nursing

Transformation theory explains how adults make sense or meaning from their experiences and has been applied successfully to numerous groups of adult learners across many educational settings. However, the theory has its roots in radical ideology, which prompts adult educators to use only one method in helping adult learners to learn (Wang & Sarbo, 2004). In reality, adult educators may assume different roles and use different learning and teaching methods (Grow, 1991). This is certainly true of nurse educators, not least because a variety of experiences and contexts, both as a practising nurse and as a nurse educator, are brought to bear on the role. The contextually adapted teaching philosophies of the educator play a major role in determining what nurse educators do to help student nurses to achieve transformation and emancipation. Therefore, while transformation theory has potential to transform the nursing curriculum from one of stasis and inflexibility to one of dynamism and flexibility, in drawing on transformation theory the role of the nurse educator needs to be considered alongside the needs of the learner. As a starting point for thinking about the role of the nurse educator, Wang and Sarbo (2004) point to a number of significant points in relation to how adult educators help adult learners achieve transformative learning. These points are adapted here to guide the development of the nursing curriculum and thus contribute to sustainable nursing practice:

1. Philosophies of nurse education provide the guiding principles for teachers of nursing: these philosophies are individual and guide action.
2. Nurse educators should consider the needs of the student nurse and their individual learning styles: together with individual teacher philosophies, these factors determine how the nurse educator assumes their role and selects their teaching methods.
3. Consideration of how nurse educators help student nurses to learn (a combination of internal philosophy, understanding of the role and selection of teaching methods) is key to the process of helping student nurses to learn.
4. For student nurses to shift to a more inclusive, emancipatory, open (to ideas) and reflexive perspective requires the learner to become skilled in critical reflection.
5. The role of the nurse educator and their choice of teaching method determines the way in which the nurse educator interacts with the student nurse. Therefore, the student nurse's development towards becoming a critically reflective practitioner is dependent on the nurse educator.

The above questions are important considerations when planning for, or revalidating the nursing curriculum, as it is often the case that a small number of educators will be involved during the development phase, while a larger number are involved in subsequent delivery of the curriculum. Nurse academics involved in the early planning phase should first consider the role and expectation of those nurse academics who will subsequently be asked to deliver the curriculum. With this in mind it is important to consider the aim of nurse education and the role of the nurse educator within this. For example, Roger's (1951) argued the aim of education was to facilitate learning, and therefore the role of the teacher was that of facilitator of learning. A faciliatory approach, such as the one advocated by Roger's, requires a shift from what the teacher does to what is happening with the student. In a nursing curriculum, prescribed by the NMC, facilitation of learning may be compromised first, by nurse educators for whom the role of facilitator of learning is resisted and second, by constraints embedded within nurse education itself, including content, competencies, assessment and the need to ensure theory/practice requirements are met. In the absence of a contextually adapted philosophy, it is difficult to make curricular decisions or to set individual curriculum policy, save that prescribed by NMC standards. As a consequence, the nursing curriculum traditionally suffers from a lack of creativity in favour of standardisation, and lack of appropriate pedagogy for nurse education (Ironside, 2004).

In summary, nurse educators are often faced with the complex task of adjusting teaching to learning with little knowledge of teaching philosophies. This is compounded when nurse teachers are drawn from practice in recognition of their expertise in clinical nursing practice, but for whom expertise in education methodologies and methods may be limited, at least at the point of appointment to the role of nurse educator. Understanding the contextual philosophies of nurse educators is to understand that no single philosophy of nurse education should dominate curriculum development, for reasons that it is determined by a multitude of factors, such as learner needs, learner styles and learner motivation, which all contribute to a working philosophy of nurse education. Understanding the complex interaction of nursing students' characteristics and the personal philosophy of the nurse educator is essential to successful adoption of transformation theory in nurse education.

Transformative Learning Experiences in the Nursing Curriculum

Mezirow described two types of transformation in meaning perspective: epochal and incremental (Mezirow, 1978). An epochal transformation occurs when a learner's meaning perspective shifts very quickly (minutes or days), sometimes referred to as a 'light bulb' moment. One example in nurse education might be when a student first hears systole and diastole when recording blood pressure. This is notoriously difficult to explain to a learner as it relies on an explanation of a sound and is somewhat of a lost art with the advent of automated measurement of blood pressure (Myers et al., 2011). An incremental transformation, on the other hand, is the result of small shifts in meaning perspective over time (months or years), which lead a learner to slowly realise that a shift has occurred. An example in terms of nurse education might be a mature student coming to university later in life having previously believed the opportunity has passed by or for a student for whom coming to university represented the first experience of higher education in the family. For both students, an incremental shift incorporates a type of retrospective remembering of a time when the opportunity to study for a university degree was believed impossible, albeit for different reasons. Both epochal and incremental transformations assume there is a conscious appreciation of a shift in meaning perspective in order for it to be recognised as transformative. In other words, the learner needs to know the shift in perspective has occurred.

When thinking about transformative learning in nurse education, three key elements described by Mezirow become important, namely, disorientating dilemmas, critical reflection and rational discourse. Experiencing each of these elements or a combination of all three elements is said to be key to transformative learning and, in this sense, can be used to guide curriculum design in nurse education. These elements are described below.

Disorientating Dilemmas

Disorientating dilemmas are one type of significant stimulus that leads people to undergo a meaning perspective transformation. A disorientating dilemma is one which causes a significant level of disruption or disturbance in a person, for example, a life crisis or major life transition, although it may result as an accumulation of transformations in meaning perspectives over time (Mezirow, 1991). Disorientating dilemmas can be quite modest, for example, a new experience, which prompts the disorientated person to examine and reflect on life prior to the experience. This reflection on life may also include an examination of values, attitudes, beliefs and their underlying tacit assumptions, which Mezirow (1991) calls critical reflection and which cannot occur without the individual first experiencing a disorientating dilemma.

Critical Reflection

Critical reflection, as a key element of transformation theory, is a process whereby a person intentionally construes new meanings from an examination of an individual set of values, attitudes and beliefs. Critical reflection occurs in numerous ways and through numerous agencies and involves identifying embedded assumptions and considering these in a rational and objective manner. Critical reflection, according to Mezirow (1991) contains three main frames. The first frame for critical reflection involves *content* reflection, or reflection on *what* happens, *how* it happens and the information supporting the focus of the reflection. For example, in assessing a mentoring experience a student nurse might reflect on the available information regarding what might be expected from mentorship and whether or not the experience met with expectation. The second frame for critical reflection concerns *process* reflection, which is reflection on whether the available content is sufficient, adequate and reliable in informing the object of the critical reflection. For example, when reflecting on a mentoring experience the student nurse might reflect on where the expectation of the mentoring process came from, the reliability of the source, and on interpretation of the information. The third frame for critical reflection is *premise* reflection, which is reflection on underlying premises, beliefs and assumptions. For example, in reflecting on a mentoring experience the student nurse might reflect on the premise on which mentorship is based, whether mentorship is a suitable mode of support for student nurses in practice settings, and whether or not mentorship is supported by the organisation such that it can be enacted. Premise reflection is considered the most important in bringing about transformational change.

Within Mezirow's transformation theory a number of component parts are needed for critical reflection to take place. These are listed below but can occur in any order:

- The means to illuminate underlying belief structures, either individually or with other people.
- Detachment from beliefs in order to be objective regarding what is being reflected on.
- Perseverance in the face of ambiguity surrounding the focus of the reflection or in response to the unsettling nature of the issue.
- The ability to think rationally about the object of the reflection in order to expose and address inconsistencies and incongruences.

The final element in Mezirow's transformation theory is rational discourse, which is said to take place when critical reflection occurs with others.

Rational Discourse

Rational discourse is the medium through which transformation is promoted and developed. It is essentially different to ordinary or 'everyday' conversations, in that it is a conversation used to question authenticity, comprehensibility and/or truthfulness of what is being asserted or to question the credibility of the person making the statement. Discourse in transformative learning is said to rest on the following assumptions:

- Discourse is rational only if it facilitates understanding with another.
- Discourse is driven by objectivity.
- Discourse is open to question and discussion.
- Understanding is arrived at by weighing and measuring all supporting evidence and argument.
- The primary goal is to promote mutual understanding among participants of the discourse.

Rational discourse is the process through which critical reflection is actualised, or in other words the mechanism through which 'praxis' within critical reflection occurs. The ability for nurses to transfer the theory of critical reflection into practice is a prerequisite for contemporary nursing, where nurses are required to think logically, with openness, and to constantly question and reflect on their practice and the practice of others (Heaslip, 2008).

Types and Levels of Reflection and Their Importance for Nurse Education

Transformative learning and reflection are a manifestation of the committed professional practice of nurses in all healthcare environments and as such should be embedded within the nursing curriculum in such a way that both teachers and students are helped to understand and acquire wisdom and sagacity about nursing. Renigere (2014) provides a useful framework for thinking about types and levels of reflection in nursing, based on Mezirow's transformation theory:

Types of Reflection

- Reflection on meaning is an examination of the content or description of a problem.
- Reflection on process includes an examination of problem-solving strategies.
- Reflection on premises leads to the meaning perspective transformation.

Levels of Reflection

- Reflection—understanding that is characterised by a specific perception, meaning, behaviour or habit (thinking in action).
- Emotional reflection—understanding how one feels regarding the perceived, her/his thought or habit (thinking in action).
- Evaluative reflection—evaluation of the effectiveness of the perception, thought or habit (thinking in action).

- Judgemental reflection—evaluation of the perception, thought, behaviour, or habit (thinking in action).
- Conceptual reflection—self-reflection that can raise doubts about the fact if good, bad or appropriate concepts were used in understanding and the evaluation process.
- Psychic reflection—acknowledges that humans tend to judge and base their judgement on a limited amount of information.
- Theoretical reflection—understanding that the ability to perceive and evaluate or the habit of conceptual inadequacy lies in cultural or psychological assumptions that are taken for granted, and that explains why a personal experience is more acceptable than another perspective that uses more functional criteria of seeing, thinking or behaviour.

In summary, for reflection to be a transferable skill for nursing practice, practising nurses need to learn how to combine the skills of reflection with skills of critical thinking (Price, 2004). Some practical ideas for incorporating critical thinking into the curriculum are considered below.

Critical Thinking

Critical thinking is the ability to think, not only about positions other than one's own but to think critically about one's own position, arguments and worldview. Critical thinking is reasonable, reflective thinking, focused on deciding what to believe or to do (Ennis, 1987). In this sense, critical thinking is predicated on the ability to become critically reflective of one's own assumptions (Mezirow, 1997). Critical thinking is argued as specific to a particular discipline, depending on the content and epistemology of that discipline (Mason, 2008). Critical thinking can be conceptualised as having a reason assessment component and a critical attitude component, with the former belonging to the skills domain, while the latter belongs to a dispositions domain. As such critical thinking is fundamental to contemporary nursing practice, which requires nurses to be knowledgeable, competent, caring and compassionate.

Critical thinking often deals with opposing views and assumptions. It is a constructive and positive process, which can be informed by negative as well as positive events. In this sense the inclusion of critical thinking in the nursing curriculum carries with it a responsibility on the part of nurse educators, to acknowledge that nursing students may come to question not only nursing practice, but also the underlying assumptions on which much nursing practice is based. Critical thinking, once mastered, has the power to reveal much that remains hidden from nursing students. While in the short-term students may become disengaged from nursing, critical thinking is not discriminatory. Rather it enables the student to develop habits (thinking in action) of inquiry and a critical curiosity about society, power and inequality, which are prerequisite for modern nursing practice.

Critical thinkers in nursing are those who are skilful in the application of intellectual skills for sound reasoning. While it may take time and experience to develop the levels of critical thinking required in complex care situations, nevertheless nurse education needs to begin the process by including classroom and clinical practice activities to develop the nursing student's critical thinking skills. Exposure to scholarly and academic work, which requires the effective use of intellectual abilities and skills, should be a prerequisite to periods of increasingly complex clinical practice, whereby students are required to think through and reason about nursing, drawing on more sophisticated understandings of what it means to nurse in contemporary healthcare settings. Approaches to teaching critical thinking to students might include:

- Reading scholarly (peer reviewed) papers.
- Writing responses to scholarly papers, which consider the full range of 'critical' positions to presented arguments.
- Listening to individual and collective responses to a range of critical positions and arguments.
- Speaking critically, in a safe environment, about the range of critical positions that might possibly be taken.

The approach highlighted here is not exhaustive but serves to illustrate how critical thinking might be included in the nursing curriculum, either as a module in and of itself or as an element within modules focused on a variety of content, for example, politics of health, ethics of healthcare, health policy and organisation. Whichever approach is ultimately taken the elemental components remain the same.

In addition to critical thinking, student nurses need to develop skills in critical reading and critical writing. Critical reading encourages students to look for assumptions, key concepts and ideas, reasons and justifications, supporting examples, parallel experiences, implications and consequences and any other structural features of the written text to interpret and assess it accurately and fairly (Paul, 1990). Critical reading should be an active, intellectually engaged process, whereby the student participates in an inner dialogue with the writer. Students have a tendency to read uncritically, missing some parts, while distorting other parts, thus giving rise to unsupported and uncritical ideas.

Critical writing requires students to be able to use appropriate forms of language to arrange ideas in some relationship to each other. Accuracy and truth in expressed language is fundamental in the student's portrayal of argument, how argument is supported, and made intelligible to others, alongside the objections which can be raised to it from others points of view, and the limitations to the student's point of view. Disciplined writing requires disciplined thinking, which is in turn achieved through disciplined writing (Heaslip, 2008).

Critical listening requires the student to monitor how they are listening in order to maximise understanding of what is being said and taught in academic and practice settings. Human communication is integral to nursing courses, usually including models of communication as a taught component, in addition to practical communication with lecturers, students, practitioners and other health professionals as the programme intensifies over time. Simulation may also be used to develop the student's communication skills. Critical listening pays attention to the logic of human communication, irrespective of approaches to teaching communication skills, that is, that all communication expresses a point of view and uses some ideas and not others. As such critical listening is a prerequisite for empathetic nursing practice.

Critical speaking involves nursing students actively expressing a point of view, idea or thought, in such a way that others can grasp an in-depth understanding of the speaker's personal perspective on the issue. By monitoring verbal expression in academic and practice settings, nursing students are enabled to maximise accurate understanding of what is meant through what is said in 'open dialogue', which is in turn subject to feedback on the view expressed.

Critical thinking is integral to critical pedagogy. As such any nursing curriculum, which takes as its starting point a critical pedagogical approach, acknowledges what Paulo Freire called conscientisation, or critical consciousness. The process of conscientisation involves identifying contradictions in experience through dialogue and becoming part of the process of changing the world (Freire, 1972). The cumulative effects of developing critical thinking skills through critical reading critical writing, critical listening and critical speaking necessarily lead to a process of conscientisation. Mechanisms for developing critical writing, reading and thinking within the nursing curriculum are covered in Chap. 5.

Conclusion

Changes to the health of populations, including increased longevity, increased long-term conditions and complex care needs, have placed a burden on governments since the inception of the NHS to find ways to meet the growing cost of an ideological commitment to universal healthcare. Technological advances in medicine including diagnosis and to an increasing extent the impact of the human genome project have seen an exponential demand for ever more technological treatment and the expectation, not just for early diagnosis and subsequent treatment but for pre-diagnostic screening for serious genetic conditions, which were previously unavailable.

Nurse education is likewise impacted by societal, healthcare, technological, economic and political factors, all of which affect the capacity for nurse education to meet its aspirational goal to prepare an educated workforce capable of working in rapidly changing healthcare contexts. Nurse education does not develop in a vacuum, independent of the wider context of health policy and organisation of health services. On the contrary, nurse education should be pedagogically responsive to these influences as it seeks to prepare students for the workplace.

However, nurse education now faces a crisis of identity, which is in part a result of failure on the part of the NMC to delineate a regulatory function from an educational function. A preoccupation with standards and competencies, while not without some justification given the recent criticisms of nurse education, nevertheless stifles creativity and innovation in curriculum development. Nurse educators need the intellectual freedom to rethink appropriate pedagogy for nursing, as a means to address the current concerns surrounding the National Health Service and to ensure nurse education is shaped in ways which recognise the need for regulation of the nursing workforce while not being subservient to it.

The following chapter considers transformative pedagogies for nurse education, in particular critical pedagogy combined with constructivist approaches to developing appropriate nursing content. Combining critical and constructivist pedagogies is argued to address concerns around the perceived failure of nurse education to educate nurses in fundamental and highly complex technical skills while at the same time delivering care with compassion in complex ethical and moral situations. The chapter develops ideas around critical writing, reading and thinking skills and mechanisms by which these can be incorporated into the nursing curriculum.

References

Campbell, D. (2016). NHS hospitals in England reveal £2.45 bn record deficit. Retrieved from http://www.theguardian.com/society/2016/may/20/nhs-in-england-reveals-245bn-record-deficit

Coles, T. (2014). Critical pedagogy: Schools must equip students to challenge the status quo. Retrieved December 13, 2016, from https://www.theguardian.com/teacher-network/teacher-blog/2014/feb/25/critical-pedagogy-schools-students-challenge

Denscombe, M. (2008). Communities of practice: A research paradigm for the mixed methods approach. *Journal of Mixed Methods Research, 2*(3), 270–283.

Dewey, J. (1938). Experience and education. Retrieved December 13, 2016, from http://ruby.fgcu.edu/courses/ndemers/colloquium/experienceeducationdewey.pdf

Eaton, A. (2012). Pre-registration nurse education: A brief history. Retrieved December 8, 2016, from www.williscommission.org.uk

Ennis, R. H. (1987). Critical thinking and the curriculum. In M. Heiman & J. Slominanko (Eds.), *Thinking skills instruction: Concepts and techniques*. Washington, DC: National Education Association.

Francis, R. (2013). *Report of the Mid Staffordshire NHS Foundation Trust public inquiry*. London: The Stationery Office.

Freire, P. (1972). *Pedagogy of the oppressed*. London: Penguin Books.

Freire, P. (1985). Reading the world and reading the word: An interview with Paulo Freire. *Language Arts, 62*(1), 15–21.

Giroux, H. A. (2011). *On critical pedagogy*. New York: Bloomsbury.

Gov.UK. (2014). Guidance: Future of apprenticeships in England: Guidance for trailblazers. Department for Business, Innovation & Skills and Department for Education. Retrieved from https://www.gov.uk/government/publications/future-of-apprenticeships-in-england-guidance-for-trailblazers

Grow, G. O. (1991). Cited in Wang, V. C. X., & Sarbo, L. (2004). Philosophy, role of adult educators, and learning. How contextually adapted philosophies and the situational role of adult educators affect learners' transformation and emancipation. *Journal of Transformative Education, 2*(3): 204–214.

Heaslip, P. (2008). Critical thinking and nursing. Retrieved May 9, 2017, from http://www.criticalthinking.org/pages/critical-thinking-and-nursing/834

Hicks, S. (2004). *Explaining postmodernism: Skepticism and socialism from Rousseau to Foucault* (pp. 18–19). Tempe, AZ: Scholargy Press.

Hughes, A. J., & Fraser, D. M. (2011). "SINK or SWIM": The experience of newly qualified midwives in England. *Midwifery, 27*(3), 382–386.

Ironside, P. M. (2001). Creating a research base for nursing education: An interpretive review of conventional, critical, feminist, postmodern, and phenomenologic pedagogies. *Advances in Nursing Science, 23*(3), 72–87.

Ironside, P. M. (2004). "Covering content" and teaching thinking: Deconstructing the additive curriculum. *Journal of Nursing Education, 43*(1), 5–12.

Kuhn, T. (1970). *The structure of scientific revolutions*. Chicago: University of Chicago Press.

Lave, J., & Wenger, E. (1991). *Situated learning: Legitimate peripheral participation*. Cambridge: Cambridge University Press.

Maguire, D., Dunn, P., & Mckenna, H. (2016). How hospital activity in the NHS in England has changed over time. Retrieved May 3, 2017, from https://www.kingsfund.org.uk/publications/hospital-activity-funding-changes

Mason, M. (2008). *Critical thinking and learning.* Oxford: Blackwell Publishing.

McLaren, P. (2009). Critical pedagogy: A look at the major concepts. In A. Darder, M. P. Baltodarno, & R. D. Torres (Eds.), *The critical pedagogy reader* (2nd ed.). New York: Routledge.

McLean, M. (2008). *Pedagogy and the university: Critical theory and practice.* London: Continuum.

Mezirow, J. (1978). Perspective transformation. *Adult Education, 28*(2), 100–110.

Mezirow, J. (1991). *Transformative dimensions of adult learning.* San Francisco: Jossey Bass.

Mezirow, J. (1997). Transformative learning: Theory to practice. *New Directions for Adult and Continuing Education, 74*, 5–12.

Myers, M. G., Godwin, M., Kiss, A., Tobe, S., Curry Grant, F., & Kaczorowski, J. (2011). Conventional versus automated measurement of blood pressure in primary care patients with systolic hypertension: Randomised parallel design controlled trial. *BMJ, 342*, d286. doi:10.1136/bmj.d286

NMC. (2010). *Standards for pre-registration nursing education.* London: NMC.

NMC. (2013). NMC response to the Francis report. The response of the Nursing and Midwifery Council to the Mid Staffordshire NHS Foundation Trust Public Inquiry report. 18 July 2016. Retrieved December 7, 2016, from http://www.nmc.org.uk/globalassets/sitedocuments/francis-report/nmc-response

Nurses, Midwives and Health Visitors Act. (1979). London: The Stationery Office.

O'Kane, C. E. (2012). Newly qualified nurses' experiences in the intensive care unit. *Nursing in Critical Care, 17*(1), 44–51.

Orton, S. (2011). Re-thinking attrition in student nurses. *Journal of Health and Social Care Improvement., 2011*, 1–7.

Pagnucci, N., Carnevale, F., Bagnasco, A., & Sasso, L. F. (2015). A Cross-sectional study of pedagogical strategies in nursing education: Opportunities and constraints toward using effective pedagogy. *BMC Medical Education, 15*, 138.

Paul, R. (1990). *Critical thinking: What every person needs to survive in a rapidly changing world.* Rohnert Park, CA: Center for Critical Thinking and Moral Critique.

Peate, I. (2013). *The student nurse toolkit: An essential guide to surviving your course.* Chichester: John Wiley and Sons Ltd.

Price, A. (2004). Encouraging reflection and critical thinking in practice. *Nursing Standard, 18*(47), 46–52.

Renigere, R. (2014). Transformative learning in the discipline of nursing. *American Journal of Educational Research, 2*(12), 1207–1210.

Report of the Committee on Nursing. (1972). Chairman: Professor Asa Briggs, Cmnd. 5115, HMSO, London.

The Cavendish Review. (2013). *An independent review into healthcare assistants and support workers in the NHS and social care settings.* London: Department of Health.

Wang, V. C. X., & Sarbo, L. (2004). Philosophy, role of adult educators, and learning: How contextually adapted philosophies and the situational role of adult educators affects learners' transformation and emancipation. *Journal of Transformative Education, 2*(3), 204–214.

WHO. (2009). *Global standards for the initial education of professional nurses and midwives.* Geneva: World Health Organisation.

5

Transforming Nurse Education

Introduction

Previous chapters have argued while developments in nurse education have attempted to address criticisms of the nursing profession, in particular a reported lack of care and compassion, nursing pedagogy has not been fully considered for its role in ensuring nurses are not only competent practitioners but are equipped with the skills necessary for critical awareness, socially conscious practice and cognitive and affective understanding of the social, political and technological context of healthcare practice. This chapter moves beyond the rhetoric in suggesting nurse educators have a responsibility to ensure nursing programmes are designed and delivered in ways, which maximise the potential for nursing students to develop the attributes necessary for present-day, modern nursing. To this end consideration is given to the role of the hidden curriculum, whereby nursing students are often left to internalise professional values consistent with nursing practice, as opposed to explicit consideration within the curriculum, so much so that the theory/practice gap persists in nursing and is of perennial concern for nursing students. The chapter considers the need for the nursing curriculum to draw on different types of nursing knowledge, in order to illuminate aspects of nursing traditionally hidden from students, but which are key to helping students to bridge the theory/practice gap, in other words to make sense of contemporary nursing practice. One such approach is a theory of constructivism, which entails a nursing curriculum predicated on the belief that individuals are able to construct their own understanding and knowledge of the world, through experiencing and reflecting on experiences. Constructivism encourages students to constantly assess how each learning activity is assisting their understanding. When used in combination with critical pedagogy nurse education becomes crucial in creating agents of change. The spiral curriculum described by Bruner (1960) is argued as one way for combining constructivism with critical pedagogy. The final section in this chapter expands on the principles of co-production first discussed in Chap. 2, paying attention to its application to nurse education. Co-creation and co-design are argued as more appropriate concepts when thinking about developing the nursing curriculum, in that their use ensures the full range of activities are encompassed, as opposed to a focus on the end point or outcome.

Nurse educators are required to maintain registration with the NMC, and as such are de facto gatekeepers of the profession. The requirement to adhere strictly to NMC standards for education determines the nature and shape of the nursing curriculum in ways often counterproductive to transformative learning, which is designed to help students find their own voice, to feel empowered to effect social change and to bring about justice for the recipients of their learning, through socially conscious practice. Nursing curricula, for the most part, adopt a model of education, which positions the teacher as expert, which focuses on subject matter, and in which information is organised in sequenced topics and units revisited over time and in increasing levels of complexity. In models of nurse education such as this, students are often not encouraged to question their own assumptions, or those of the teacher. This conventional approach to the nursing curriculum considers the teachers experience as most valuable for providing insight, which thus determines the teachers understanding of what knowledge and skills the students need to have, the assumption being that both knowledge of and experience of nursing practice can be transferred to students simply by transmitting information, as opposed to transforming student thinking.

In contrast to conventional approaches to nurse education, the desired outcome of nursing curricula underpinned by transformative pedagogy is to change, to transfer learning into social action outside the classroom and into the world of nursing work. Teachers engaged in transformative pedagogy relinquish notions of teacher as holder of knowledge to one where students need to create knowledge for themselves.

Transformative pedagogy places the student at the centre of learning. Teachers, engaged in transformative pedagogy empower students through appropriate teaching methods to effect change in nursing practice. Students come to know, not only how to practise nursing but how to understand nursing practice. While most nurse educators understand the goal of nurse education in this sense, nevertheless current approaches to nurse education inhibit the joint construction of knowledge, required for learning to be transferred effectively from classroom to the practice setting. Transformative pedagogy, on the other hand, incorporates and builds on notions of critical pedagogy, paying attention to underlying concepts of the hidden curriculum. While the concept of the hidden curriculum is not new, having been first muted by Paulo Freire, nevertheless the concept is relevant to contemporary nurse education, in so much as it places emphasis on those unstated values, norms and attitudes, which stem tacitly from the social relations of the learning setting, in addition to the content of the nursing programme.

The Hidden Curriculum in Nursing

The formal nursing curriculum involves all the aspects that make up the whole, including philosophical approaches, curriculum outcomes, overall design, modules, units or courses, learning and teaching strategies, delivery methods, student-teacher relationships, evaluation processes and resources (Karimi, Ashktourab, Mohammadi, & Ali Abedi, 2014). However, a curriculum is more than a syllabus or statement of intent, being as much about what is often covert or hidden, as opposed to overtly or explicitly stated. The hidden curriculum operates at organisational, structural and cultural levels, covering a set of unwritten social and cultural values, rules, assumptions and expectations, which impact more strongly on the recipients, compared to the formal curriculum.

Professionalism in nursing is traditionally the part of the hidden curriculum, understood and 'caught' or internalised, rather than explicitly taught, with emphasis given to teaching core competencies and psychomotor skills. Nursing students may subsequently be left to internalise professional values consistent with nursing practice—altruism, autonomy, human dignity, integrity and social justice (Shaw & Degazon, 2008), as opposed to externalising professional values in the workplace. A side effect of implicitly, as opposed to explicitly teaching professionalism results in students who are technically competent, but deficient in the skills needed to effect change and to influence nursing practice.

The hidden curriculum, whose function includes the inculcation of values, political socialisation, and training in obedience and docility (Vallance, 1983), may in part be responsible for disenfranchisement of nurses, who are subsequently unable to challenge poor practice, to advocate on behalf of patients and to defend the rights of patients to expect the highest standards of care. While the nursing curriculum may include a theoretical component on professionalism, for example, role modelling, leadership, ethics and ways of thinking about nursing, internalisation of professionalism is often left to the students themselves, resulting in dissonance between theory and practice, when students are later exposed to the clinical environment. Inconsistencies between theory and practice have potential to challenge students with complicated, emotional and ethical problems. This theory-practice gap is of perennial concern to students and educators and arises in part from the hidden curriculum. Students are often taught an idealised version of nursing, which cannot be accommodated in the real-life social settings in which nursing work occurs. Students, and nurse educators for that matter, may understand the nursing curriculum in a rhetorical sense, nevertheless a curriculum is not fully understood unless the hidden curriculum is taken into consideration. Students need exposure to the developmental history of the profession, to the relationship of professional roles, one with another, and to the current cultural, sociological and political influences on practice in order to prepare them for nursing leadership, in addition to preparation for nursing proficiency. In other words, nursing students need to be prepared in both the art and the science of nursing. The nursing curriculum needs to draw on different types of nursing knowledge, to ensure aspects of professionalism, traditionally hidden within the curriculum are made explicit and subject to critical examination.

Nursing Knowledge

The body of knowledge, drawn on by a particular discipline, is determined by how a discipline conceives of itself. Scientific disciplines are likely to draw on scientific forms of knowledge, whereas human science disciplines are likely, although not exclusively, to draw on experiential knowledge. Identification of a body of nursing knowledge has occupied the minds of nurse academics keen to develop and clarify the body of nursing knowledge (Rogers, 1989), albeit less so since nursing became recognised as an academic discipline upon moving into higher education. Nursing as a discipline is by definition complex, being considered both art and science. Nursing knowledge should underpin conceptualisation of nursing as a critical social enterprise, where issues of social justice are central to its endeavours, in addition to providing a rationale for both theory and practice components.

Nursing knowledge is thought to rest on evidence derived from scientific knowledge (knowledge developed through enquiry), experiential knowledge (knowledge gained from exposure with practice) and from personal knowledge (knowledge from prior learning), including life experiences. Understanding nursing knowledge is necessary for learning and teaching nursing that is of equal importance to teachers and students. Focusing attention on nursing knowledge involves critical attention to what forms of knowledge are valued and are *of value* to nursing.

Barbara Carper originally wrote of nursing knowledge in 1975, distinguishing four fundamental patterns of knowing according to their logical type or meaning:

1. Empirics, the science of nursing
2. Aesthetics, the art of nursing

3. The component of personal knowledge in nursing
4. Ethics, the component of moral knowledge in nursing

With respect to empirics or the science of nursing, Carper noted the term *nursing science* was rarely used in the literature until the late 1950s, after which time a sense of urgency accompanied an increasing emphasis regarding the development of a body of empirical knowledge specific to nursing. The pattern of knowing generally designated as nursing science was thought not to exhibit the same degree of highly integrated abstract and systematic explanations characteristic of the more mature sciences. Nursing literature at that time tended towards discussing the concept of nursing science as an 'ideal form', of most importance, should nursing wish to be considered a profession in its own right and not simply allied to medicine. For Carper, the first fundamental pattern of knowing in nursing is empirical, factual, descriptive and ultimately aimed at developing abstract and theoretical explanations.

When discussing aesthetics, the art of nursing, Carper implicitly criticised the professional nursing literature for focusing on the development of nursing science to the detriment of the aesthetic pattern of knowing in nursing, other than to vaguely associate the *art of nursing* with the general category of manual and/or technical skills involved in nursing practice. In this sense Carper was ahead of her time in conceptualising nursing as more than a practical endeavour, in which mastery of skills designated as 'nursing work' defined nursing, to the exclusion of other forms of nursing knowledge. This reluctance to acknowledge the aesthetic component as a fundamental pattern of knowing in nursing, she said,

> originates in the vigorous efforts made in the not-so-distant past to exorcise the image of the apprentice-type educational system. Within the apprentice system, the art of nursing was closely associated with an imitative learning style and the acquisition of knowledge by accumulation or unrationalized experiences. (Carper, 1978, p. 26)

Efforts to distance nursing from apprenticeship style training led nursing theorists to disengage with ideas that nursing draws on forms of knowledge other than knowledge gained by empirical description.

However, in more recent times, following implied criticism of nursing practice, and by implication of nurse education, the acquisition of empirical nursing knowledge has taken precedence over aesthetic nursing knowledge. The public, the media and government are concerned less with the 'art of nursing' and more with the science of nursing. Although not expressed directly as a call for the return of an *apprenticeship model*, nevertheless nurse education is often criticised for its place in the academy. In the wake of the Francis Inquiry, the locale for nurse education has taken centre stage, as opposed to re-considering appropriate forms of nursing knowledge underpinning nursing pedagogy.

Nursing as 'art and science' includes personal knowledge in nursing. Carper acknowledged this was the most difficult component to teach, while at the same time being the pattern most essential to understanding the meaning of health in terms of individual well-being. Nursing, according to Carper is considered an interpersonal process involving interactions, relationships, and transactions between nurses and patients/clients. Nursing requires nurses to be alert to the fact that models of human nature and their abstract and generalised categories refer to and describe behaviours and traits that groups have in common. However, none of these categories can ever encompass or express the uniqueness of the individual encountered person, as a 'self'. Hence the need for a pedagogy of nursing, to encompass a constructivist component to enable students to achieve competency in nursing practice, and critical pedagogy to enable students to critically question nursing practice, and the theories on which practice is based.

The ethical component of nursing knowledge pays attention to the different personal choices that must be made within the context of modern healthcare. Contemporary healthcare practice, which emphasises choice in terms of individual access to treatment, and location of service delivery, implies the equitable distribution of personal and organisation resources, and assumes a level of knowledge supported by advances in technology. However, the fair and impartial distribution of resources, as an espoused goal of the NHS, is not borne out in reality, with wide variations reported in the UK with respect to early diagnoses of cancer, access to emergency care, major disparities in dementia care, access to timely treatment for stroke or treatment for many common health complaints such as treatment for cataracts (NHS Atlas of Variation in Healthcare, 2015). The ethical component of nursing knowledge focuses on matters of obligation for nurses, or what ought to be done, for example a consideration of social inequalities in health, socially unfair health practices, issues of discrimination, unfair treatment, stereotyping, abusive practice and bullying.

The moral component of nursing knowledge allows nursing students to reconcile nursing as a deliberate action, or series of actions, planned and implemented to accomplish defined goals, in part on the basis of normative judgement. On occasion the principles and norms by which such choices are made may give rise to conflict between nurse and patient, patient and healthcare provider, nurse and doctor and nursing student and nursing lecturer. Carper's work on nursing knowledge, although of its time, provided the means for an increased awareness of the complexity and diversity of nursing knowledge, which is as relevant today as when first postulated.

More recently, Cipriano (2007) has described five ways of knowing, useful in understanding how one comes to know or have knowledge of something: empirical knowing, ethical knowing, personal knowing, aesthetic knowing and finally synthesising, which pulls together knowledge gained from the four types of knowledge. The parallels with Carper's earlier work are clear to see. Modern nursing requires nurse educators to design nursing curricula predicated on an understanding of nursing as art, as science, as an ethical and moral endeavour, and as a personal commitment. Understanding nursing knowledge in this way enables nurse educators to conceptualise a nursing curriculum, in which constructivism and critical pedagogy can be used in combination to transform nursing pedagogy.

It is clear that nursing knowledge encompasses aspects of knowledge, which are of relevance to nursing (Edwards, 2002). However, it is important to note the types of knowledge drawn on by nursing vary over time, being influenced by contextual factors impacting nursing at a given moment, for example the changing political landscape in which health and social care services are delivered. In essence, this requires nurse educators charged with developing the nursing curriculum to go beyond traditional ways of understanding nursing to redefine nursing knowledge, which then needs to be constructed within the curriculum.

Constructivism in Nurse Education

Constructivism in education is concerned with how students learn best. A constructivist view of learning assumes individuals are able to construct their own understanding and knowledge of the world, through experiencing and reflecting on experiences. In the classroom setting, constructivist approaches generally adopt active teaching styles, for example problem-based learning, as these are thought to create knowledge, which students can then reflect on. Constructivist teaching requires the teacher to encourage the learner to engage in constant assessment of how each learning activity is assisting their understanding; the idea being that constant questioning enables students to become expert learners, transferable across time and settings.

Constructivist approaches to curriculum development are often manifest within the spiral curriculum, first postulated by Jerome Bruner in 1960. In a spiral curriculum information is reinforced and solidified each time the learner revisits the subject matter. A spiral curriculum thus allows for logical progression from simplistic ideas to complicated ideas, with learners encouraged to apply early knowledge to later course objectives. Constructivist teaching within a spiral curriculum may work well where learners need to become familiar with a set of practices or concepts, which remain relatively stable. For example, those concepts considered to underpin nursing practice, treating people with dignity and respect, taking responsibility for one's own judgement and actions, managing risk, and maintaining safety, promoting patient-centred care, communicating effectively, and keeping up to date with new knowledge and skills. Nursing students will revisit these concepts, in addition to continuous exposure to practical skills teaching and continuous experience in practice settings, throughout the nursing curriculum. The concept of the spiral curriculum is thought to have educational value, in that an iterative revisiting of topics, subjects, themes and concepts, at deepening levels of complexity enables students to relate new learning to old learning, thus increasing student competency (Smith, 2002).

Nursing curricula, underpinned by a spiral design, builds learning progressively, with the idea that students will be enabled, at the end of the nursing programme, to see nursing as a whole, in other words to fit the pieces of the nursing puzzle together. The assumption made, however, is that first, students have retained previously learned material (Masters & Gibbs, 2007), and second that students have not only assimilated the material but are able to think critically around the information, in ways which will enable transference of learning to increasingly complex settings, or, as is often the case, increasingly uncertain practice environments. A spiral curriculum, underpinned by constructivist approaches to learning and teaching requires the addition of critical pedagogy in order to become a transformative pedagogy, with potential to empower students to critically examine their beliefs, values and knowledge with the goal of developing a reflective knowledge base, an appreciation of multiple perspectives, and a sense of critical consciousness and agency (Ukpokodu, 2009).

When combined with constructivist approaches to teaching competency for practice, for example problem-based learning techniques, the addition of critical pedagogy provides for a curriculum, which addresses the broader scope and vision of nurse education, resulting in a nursing curriculum with potential to transform nurse education and nursing practice. Critical pedagogy is thus a transformative pedagogy, which, when used to underpin the nursing curriculum brings nursing students to a level of consciousness about nursing, in preparation for the realities of nursing practice.

Critical Pedagogy in Nursing

Applying critical pedagogy to nursing requires nurse educators to first see education as a crucial foundation for creating agents of change, who can live in, govern and influence healthcare decision-making at the level of government, and within organisations internationally, nationally and locally. Second, nurse educators need to understand education as a moral and political practice, which carries with it a social responsibility to educate nursing students, not just towards achievement of NMC defined clinical competencies and knowledge to underpin competent practice, but also for the rigours of contemporary nursing practice. In essence nursing programmes should provide nursing students with the knowledge and skills to enable them to be engaged critical citizens, willing to advocate on behalf of patients and clients and able to stand up and speak up for those whose voices are often not heard.

The vision and mission of nursing programmes must extend beyond preparing nurses who are described as fit for purpose and for practice, but where nursing is defined by government and its associated organisations and institutions. Nurses need to be enabled, through initial education programmes, to take the lead in defining what nursing practice should look like, to examine the deficiencies in current models of healthcare delivery, and to take a leading role in transforming the workplace for the mutual benefit of patients and clients. All healthcare professionals strive to provide high-quality care with compassion. However, healthcare professionals, including nurses, have the right to work in safe conditions, conducive to lifelong learning. Nurse educators need to understand their role as not about protecting the borders of the nursing curricula in order to perpetuate a "professionalised gated community" (Giroux, 2006, p. 64) but to preserve the critically socially conscious culture that can support nursing students to develop knowledge, discernment and socially critical skills necessary for a client-centred healthcare system.

It is the responsibility of all nurse educators to shape nurse education into environments, which maximise the potential for nursing students to become agents for transformational change in nursing practice. Thoughtful approaches to nursing pedagogy and curriculum design, which recognise nurse education as more than simply preparing a student to be fit for a purpose, defined by politicians and policy makers, should be the fundamental aspiration of nurse education. While standards, protocols and competencies are ways of ensuring basic minimum standards are met, it is worth noting that the problems at Mid Staffordshire NHS Foundation Trust happened *after* the world of standards, protocols and competencies and not before. Nurse educators must ask what the place of critical pedagogy is in what has come to be known inappropriately and unhelpfully as the post-Francis era. There is a very real danger that in simply adopting the phraseology of the moment—'care and compassion'—that nurse education will systematically fail to understand how students learn and how nursing students learn to care. Nurses need to not only adopt a critical stance towards nursing practice, but also to think critically about nurse education.

Transformative Pedagogy

Pedagogy at its most fundamental level refers to the art and science of being a teacher, being concerned with strategies and styles of teaching. Transformative pedagogy transcends this fundamental understanding of pedagogy through emphasis on multiple perspectives on the learning and teaching experience (Mezirow, 1997). Transformative pedagogy refers to interactional processes and dialogues between educators and students, which invigorate the collaborative creation and distribution of power in the learning setting (Salama, 2009).

Transformative pedagogy within nursing education involves reconciling the creation of ideas and solutions, with the social and environmental responsibilities embedded within the art, science and ethical and moral aspects of nursing. By this is meant the importance of assisting students to understand the current context in which NHS services are delivered, the mechanisms at play within it, including the political context, while at the same time encouraging students to be creative, find solutions to issues, and more importantly to understand what can be accepted in terms of care delivery and what should not be tolerated.

Within the context of nursing education, learners construct knowledge in educational and practice settings, making it imperative for pedagogical approaches within the nursing curriculum, which facilitate the transference of learning from one setting to the other, thus enabling students to think critically and to critically question nursing knowledge in all its forms. Transformative pedagogy is an activist pedagogy, which combines elements of constructivism, whereby students construct knowledge through interaction with the learning environment, and critical pedagogy, which enables nursing students to question and challenge dominant positions (Ukpokodu, 2009).

Transformative pedagogy, which combines critical pedagogy and constructivist pedagogy, is an appropriate pedagogical approach for nurse education, in that it is realist pedagogy, based on contemporary, while at the same time possible, pathways with the ultimate goal of improving the experience of patients, families and carers. In addition, a transformative pedagogical approach to the nursing curriculum, in theory and in practice, mitigates tension between the requirement to prepare competent nurses, with the need to prepare nurses with the skills to not only to construct the world around them, but to impact the world around them. Co-production provides the means through which transformative pedagogical approaches can be enacted in the nursing curriculum.

Co-production in Education

Co-production, as we have seen in Chap. 2, has its roots in the work of Elinor Ostrom and colleagues, later built upon through the work of Edgar Cahn to rethink the design and delivery of health and social care services to better include the views of service users. Co-production refers to active input by people who use services, as well as, or instead of, those who have traditionally provided them, and is most often associated with public service delivery, particularly adult social care. Co-production principles recognise people are not passive recipients of services but have assets and expertise that can improve services. In this sense co-production is a transformative way of thinking about power, resources, partnerships, risks and outcomes. The concept of co-production applies equally well to education, as it relates to the generation of social capital—the reciprocal relationship that builds trust, peer support and social activism among communities (Needham, 2009). Social capital is an important concept within educational settings, being thought to improve both student experience and student performance.

The original idea of social capital in education is credited to American philosopher, psychologist and educational reformer John Dewey, whose early ideas about the importance of individuals associating with one another led him to use the term social capital in 1900, when explaining the importance of reading, writing and arithmetic to the social life of the student. Dewey believed these subjects were social in a double sense. First, they represented the tools which society has evolved in the past as the instruments of its intellectual pursuits, and second, they represent the keys to unlock to the child the wealth of social capital, which lies beyond the possible range of his limited experience (Dewey, cited by Plagens, 2011). Social capital has since been considered as a multidimensional concept, where group membership provides benefits to members, which might otherwise be unavailable. Eleanor Ostrom, the pioneering thinker around co-production argued that social capital is human made, in the same manner as physical and human capital are human made (Ostrom, 1996). All three forms, physical, human and social capital, grow out of transaction and transformation activities. Individuals, she argues, build social capital when they spend time and effort taking a set of physical inputs and transforming them into another set, which may be used in further transformation activity, with the former referring to the relationships among the individuals involved in the process and the latter referring to the process itself. Social capital has come to be understood as describing the pattern and intensity of networks among people and the shared values which arise from those networks (ONS, 2016). Higher levels of social capital are associated with better health and higher educational attainment. Social capital in education is considered in Dewey's original work and in the later work by Ostrom as a process of transformation, whereby more senior members of society interact with younger members, and as a result transmit from one generation to the next what is deemed necessary to achieve desired results.

Social Capital in Nurse Education

The concept of social capital is an important one for nurse education, in the sense that nursing students become part of a community of practice, which encompasses theoretical and practice settings, and in which the aims, beliefs, aspirations and knowledge, in other words, a common understanding of nursing are shared. The norms and values of nursing are transmitted to the learner nurse through engagement with these communities of practice. The ability of the communities of practice to convey strong norms of nursing, for example respecting individual choice, respect for privacy and dignity, and recognition of one's own limitations, determine whether the social capital generated works to the advantage or disadvantage of the learner. Not all norms are positive. In situations, such as those occurring at Mid Staffordshire NHS Foundation Trust, 'the norm' became one where the rights of patients, families and carers were consistently ignored (Francis, 2013). The failure of the communities of practice to convey strong positive norms of nursing practice impacts the capacity for nurses and nursing students to accrue social capital, which in turn increases the likelihood of individual action as opposed to collective action. Bourdieu argues "social capital is the sum of the resources, actual or virtual, that accrue to an individual or a group by virtue of possessing a durable network of more or less institutionalised knowledge of mutual acquaintance and recognition" (Bourdieu, in Bourdieu & Wacquant, 1992, p. 119). This darker view of social capital goes some way towards explaining why nurses at the hospital felt unable to 'speak out'. In this sense, social capital can be a force binding people together in ways which can be exclusionary and ultimately damaging.

A framework of questions with supporting rationale, derived from Plagens (2011) work on social capital and education is set out below. The framework can be used to prompt nurse educators to identify opportunities for students to accrue social capital within nursing programmes. Communities of practice are considered in this framework to include all settings where nursing is taught and practiced. Question one asks:

> *What opportunities are provided within the nursing curriculum for student volunteering?*

Plagens argues that individuals in high social capital communities have learned to be more socially cooperative. This is not to say that individuals do not possess personal interests; it is certain they do. However, those interests do not prevent them from working with others towards a common purpose. When action is required for the benefit of the community, socially cooperative individuals are likely to participate in the process. Plagens suggests individuals may have acquired this trait through transgenerational norms, through the efforts of cooperatively minded individuals to establish such a norm, or through participation in network activity. Social cooperation within nursing is an important concept. Nurses are expected to develop professional relationships with practitioners, clinicians, healthcare managers and policy makers. Deficiencies in collaboration and communication between healthcare professionals have a negative impact on the provision of healthcare and on patient outcomes (Martin, Ummenhofer, Manser, & Spirig, 2010).

Nursing students engage with others through a variety of relationships, forming many different types of networks. Social capital is the resource that stems from these social interactions, networks and network opportunities which take place in specific environments (Boeck et al., 2009). Providing nursing students with opportunities for volunteering, either as part of the formal nursing programme or as an extra-curricular activity, can help establish norms of social cooperation necessary for effective nursing practice.

Question two asks:

> *How does the nursing curriculum encourage student nurses to take an interest in and have knowledge of the community (locally and more broadly) and its issues?*

Nurses serve as significant knowledge brokers within healthcare systems, among healthcare disciplines and with patients, families and communities. Where individuals take an interest in and have knowledge of the community and its issues, there is likely to be a norm reinforcing such behaviour and active networks facilitating the spread of knowledge (Plagens, 2011). While traditional ways of introducing nursing students to communitarian issues might predominate within the curriculum, nevertheless as technology rapidly advances, so too should pedagogy in nurse education. Understanding how technology can provide a medium for learning and teaching, outside the traditional classroom is increasingly important for the future of nurse education (Schmitt, Sims-Giddens, & Booth, 2012). Creating a professional voice, and enhancing engagement with wider social issues affecting communities, through expansion of technological abilities are critical skills for nursing students. Nurse educators need to explore the possibilities offered by social media platforms to engage students with communities while taking account of policy, privacy, time, cost, risk and lack of familiarity with technology for both teachers and students. Question three requires nurse educators to consider:

> *How does the nursing curriculum promote solidarity and genuine feelings of care about the community of practice?*

Genuine care about community issues is likely to result in community-enhancing behaviour (Plagens, 2011). Strong feelings of genuine concern are thought one reason that communities are likely to provide services to those who they believe are unable or incapable of caring or providing for themselves. Implicit within nursing's community of practice is a 'norm of solidarity', which helps explain why nurses feel genuine concern for patients, clients, families, carers and other healthcare professionals. Paying attention to curriculum content around the politics of health, including, for example, the equitable distribution of scarce health resources, equal access to timely diagnosis, best treatment, and local access to healthcare services assists students to not only gain a wider understanding of issues affecting communities but also how they relate to communities on an individual level. Including content such as this within the curriculum helps develop norms prohibiting inward facing behaviours, in favour of behaviours consistent with the philosophy of nursing. Question four is concerned with:

> *How does the nursing curriculum assist nursing students to build positive identification with the community of practice?*

Individuals in high social capital communities are more likely to identify with the community of practice and to view this identity favourably. In recent times, however, nursing and nurse education has been subject to criticism by the public, by the media, and by government. The phrase 'too posh to wash' has been used as a derogation of nurses who are now educated to degree level (Hall, 2004). The publication of the report of the public inquiry into the Mid Staffordshire NHS Foundation Trust and why its failures were not recognised sooner by the wider NHS is considered a pivotal point in nursing's recent history, such that it is considered the most important look at the NHS, and by implication at nursing for at least 20 years. The failings identified by the Francis Inquiry are not the only place where concerns have been raised. Maidstone and Winterbourne View are two further examples of devastating failures in care, so much so that nursing as a profession has seen a lack of confidence and trust in the profession (2020 Health, 2013). Nurse educators have a role to play in ensuring nursing students positively identify with nursing as a profession. Feelings of positive identification lead to participation in existing networks, and to build and maintain reciprocal relationships with other students, with teachers, and professional nurses. Encouraging student nurses to engage with networks, for example, the Royal College of Nursing and the National Union of Students (NUS), can do much to promote a positive image of nursing and go some way towards regaining the trust of the public in the profession of nursing. Finally, question five considers:

> How are nursing students assisted to develop trust in the community of practice and in each other?

Individuals in solidaristic communities will be much more likely to trust others in their community (Plagens, 2011). Trust, however, is a much-debated concept. Whether individuals come to trust others because they interact with them or whether they interact with others because they are predisposed to trust in not clear. Nevertheless, nursing is predicated on being able to 'trust' on many levels, for example, patients need to trust nurses, nurses need to trust healthcare organisation management, and student nurses need to trust that nurse education will provide them with the tools and skills required for contemporary nursing practice. In education and practice settings student nurses who trust lecturers and mentors are more likely to communicate issues, which might impact performance. One way of conceptualising trust is to think of it as the mutual experiences and obligations that participating parties, that is students, teachers, mentors, expect of one another in the community of practice (Bryk & Schneider, 2002). For example, students expect that teachers and mentors will take the necessary actions to help them achieve programme outcomes. Teachers expect students to engage with the nursing programme, inclusive of theory and practice elements, in ways consistent with norms of professional behaviour. Each party trusts that the other will do their part. Any lapse in obligation reduces the quality of the relationship among the constituent parties, creating disharmony and problems, which impede progress towards programme goals. Paying attention to issues of trust in nursing programmes assists nurse educators to consider how assessment processes, including feedback on performance, written or practical, is communicated and how opportunities for improving performance are managed (Killingley & Dyson, 2016).

The questions suggested here are not exhaustive, but do provide a basis on which to consider opportunities within the nursing curriculum for students to accrue social capital. Describing nursing as a community of practice mitigates the false division between theory and practice. Conceptualising nursing and nurse education within a 'community of practice' recognises the shared aims, beliefs, aspirations, knowledge and common understanding of what nursing is and what it means to be a nurse in modern society.

Social capital is integral to a nursing curriculum, which recognises the value of co-productive approaches to nursing pedagogy. To reiterate Needham's (2009) view, co-production is a transformative way of thinking about power, resources, partnerships, risks and outcomes. Social capital results from a co-produced approach to nursing pedagogy. The reciprocal relationships involved in co-producing the nursing curriculum build trust, peer support and social activism among nursing's community of practice.

Co-creating the Nursing Curriculum

The NMC requires evidence that practitioners, students and service users are involved throughout curriculum development; thus, the concept of co-production is well established in nurse education while not necessarily being explicitly stated. Co-creation, as opposed to co-production, is arguably a more appropriate term to frame curriculum development, in that the concept of co-creation can be used effectively to ensure inclusivity throughout the planning and design process. Co-creation refers to any act of collective creativity that is shared by two or more people and in broad terms can range from a number of activities including thinking through the philosophical basis for the curriculum to defining and explicitly stating programme aims and objectives. Using co-creation as opposed to co-production allows for a focus on the range of activities encompassing the whole process of curriculum development, from initial planning stages, through to and including the validated curriculum, rather than a focus on the end point or outcome. Co-design, often used interchangeably with co-creation occurs when the expertise of others is recognised as important to the initial critical phase of curriculum development, as opposed to later involvement in curriculum delivery. This front end of design, whether it be a service, a product or a programme, is often characterised by ambiguity and chaos and, in this sense, has been referred to the fuzzy end of the process (Sanders & Stappers, 2008). The aim of curriculum development at this stage is to bring together many perspectives, for example, service uses with their unique understanding of healthcare services, students with their understanding of adult learning and non-nursing disciplines for transferable learning to nursing. The value of creative connections in the initial planning stages determines what should and sometimes what should not be designed.

Conclusion

This chapter has considered transformative approaches to nurse education, making the case for combining constructivism; as a means of ensuring students develop nursing competency, with critical pedagogy, as a means of ensuring students develop the abilities to critically examine nurse education and nursing practice. The role of the hidden curriculum was identified as significant in perpetuating the theory-practice gap in nursing, whereby students report what is taught in theory is often not enacted in practice. Revealing the hidden curriculum to nursing students, for example, the realities of contemporary nursing practice, is argued to mitigate the 'reality shock' often experienced by neophyte nursing students and responsible in part for high attrition from nursing programmes. Forms of knowledge, empirical, aesthetical, personal, ethical and moral, of value to, and valued in, nursing enable nursing to be conceptualised as a unique and complex discipline, as art, as science and as a personal and moral enterprise.

The chapter concluded by examining the role of co-production as a means of enacting transformative pedagogical approaches to curriculum development. Co-production, although associated with active input of users of services, as opposed to those who traditionally supply services, was suggested as equally applicable to education settings, in particular as a means of ensuring nursing students accrue social capital. Social capital is seen as integral to nursing programmes, if nurses are to develop the norms associated with nursing; the shared aims, values, beliefs and attitudes consistent with a philosophy of nursing. A framework of questions for interrogation of the nursing curriculum was suggested as a means of assessing the potential for nursing students to accrue social capital, for example, through volunteering opportunities, community engagement, positive identification with nursing as a profession and trust in each other and in members of the community of practice.

The following chapter considers how a philosophy of co-creation provides a way forward for nurse education in a post-Francis era, with examples of how a co-created curriculum might work in practice.

References

Boeck, T., Makadia, N., Johnson, C., Cadogan, N., Salim, H., & Cushing, J. (2009). The impact of volunteering on social capital and community cohesion. Retrieved July 18, 2016, from http://www.dmu.ac.uk/documents/health-and-life-sciences-documents/centre-for-social-action/research/project-reaction-final-report.pdf

Bourdieu, P., & Wacquant, L. J. D. (1992). *An invitation to reflexive sociology*. Chicago: University of Chicago Press.

Bruner, J. S. (1960). *The process of education*. Cambridge, MA: Harvard University Press.

Bryk, A. S., & Schneider, B. (2002). *Trust in schools: A core resource for improvement*. New York, NY: Russell Sage Foundation.

Carper, B. A. (1978). Fundamental patterns of knowing in nursing. *Advances in Nursing Science, 1*(1), 13–24.

Cipriano, P. (2007). Celebrating the art and science of nursing. *American Nurse Today, 2*(5), 8.

Dewey, J. (1900). The psychology of the elementary curriculum. Cited by Plagens, G. (2011). Social capital and education: Implications for student and school performance. *E&C/Education &Culture, 27*(1): 40–64.

Edwards, S. (2002). Nursing knowledge: Defining new boundaries (art and science development). *Nursing Standard, 17*(2), 40–44.

Francis, R. (2013). *Report of the Mid Staffordshire NHS Foundation Trust public inquiry*. London: The Stationery Office.

Giroux, H. A. (2006). Higher education under siege: Implications for public intellectuals. *The NEA Higher Education Journal*, Fall, 63–78.

Hall, C. (2004, May 11). Young nurses "too posh to wash". *The Telegraph*. Retrieved December 21, 2016, from http://www.telegraph.co.uk/news/uknews/1461504/Young-nurses-too-posh-to-wash.html

Karimi, Z., Ashktourab, T., Mohammadi, M., & Ali Abedi, H. (2014). Using the hidden curriculum to teach professionalism in nursing students. *Iranian Red Crescent Medical Journal, 16*(3), e15532.

Killingley, J., & Dyson, S. E. (2016). Student midwives' perspectives on efficacy of feedback after structured clinical examination. *British Journal of Midwifery, 24*(5), 362–368.

Martin, J. S., Ummenhofer, W., Manser, T., & Spirig, R. (2010). Interprofessional collaboration among nurses and physicians: Making a difference in patient outcomes. *Swiss Medical Weekly, 140*, w13062.

Masters, K., & Gibbs, T. (2007). The spiral curriculum: Implications for on-line learning. *BMC Medical Education, 7*(1), 52.

Mezirow, J. (1997). Transformative learning: Theory to practice. *New Directions for Adult and Continuing Education, 74*, 5–12.

Needham, C. (2009). SCIE Research briefing 31: Co-production: An emerging evidence base for adult social care transformation. Retrieved July 18, 2016, from http://www.scie.org.uk/publications/briefings/briefing31/

NHS Atlas of Variation in Healthcare. (2015). Retrieved from http://www.rightcare.nhs.uk/atlas/2015_IAb/atlas.html

Office for National Statistics (ONS). (2016). What works wellbeing. Retrieved July 18, 2016, from https://whatworkswellbeing.org/2016/05/26/social-capital-across-the-uk/

Ostrom, E. (1996). Crossing the great divide: Coproduction, synergy, and development. *World Development, 24*(6), 1073–1087.

Rogers, B. L. (1989). Concepts, analysis and the development of nursing knowledge: The evolutionary cycle. *Journal of Advanced Nursing, 14*, 330–335.

Salama, A. M. (2009). *Transformative pedagogy in architecture and urbanism*. Solingen: Umbau-Verlag.

Sanders, B. N., & Stappers, P. J. (2008). Co-creation and the new landscapes of design. *CoDesign, 4*(1), 5–18.

Schmitt, T., Sims-Giddens, S., & Booth, R. (2012). Social media use in nursing education. *The Online Journal of Issues in Nursing, 17*(3), 2.

Shaw, H. K., & Degazon, C. (2008). Integrating the core professional values of nursing: A profession, not just a career. *Journal of Cultural Diversity, 15*(1), 44–50.

Smith, M. K. (2002). Jerome Bruner and the process of education. *The Encyclopaedia of Informal Education*. Retrieved July 18, 2016, from http://infed.org/mobi/jerome-bruner-and-the-process-of-education/

Ukpokodu, O. N. (2009). Pedagogies that foster transformative learning in a multicultural education course: A refection. *Journal of Praxis in Multicultural Education, 4*(1). doi:10.9741/2161-2978.1003

Vallance, E. (1983). Hiding the hidden curriculum: An interpretation of the language of justification in nineteenth-century educational reform. In H. Giroux & D. Purpel (Eds.), *The hidden curriculum and moral education* (pp. 9–27). Berkeley, CA: McCutchan Publishing Corporation.

www.2020Health.org. (2013). Too Posh to Wash? Reflections on the future of nursing January 2013. Retrieved July 18, 2016, from www.2020health.org/dms/2020health/downloads/reports/2020tooposh_06-02-13

6

Co-creation in Nurse Education

Introduction

This chapter considers the philosophy of co-creation and how co-creation might work within nurse education. The chapter argues while many nurse educators engage in co-creation this is usually confined to activities at the level of the classroom, and as such is limited to learning and teaching methods, with the result that a philosophy of co-creation does not permeate curriculum development in any meaningful sense. The chapter begins by looking at the underpinning philosophy of co-creation, before considering different pragmatic approaches to developing a co-creative approach to the nursing curriculum.

Students are a key resource within nurse education for reasons that the statutory body for the regulation of nurse education in the UK, the NMC, requires students to spend 50% of their learning in the practice setting. This requirement invariably means nursing students accrue practice experience, which is often both more contextual and more current than that of the nurse educators who are teaching them. Despite this, nursing students are rarely, if ever, consulted about their educational experiences with a view to informing the nursing curriculum, although they will be assessed in practice on the achievement of clinical competency. This represents a lost opportunity to engage students in the designing of teaching approaches, courses and content, in other words co-creation of the curriculum, in ways which would harness the potential for students to move from passivity to agency, a shift which is crucial in the current context of the NHS.

The notion of the co-created curriculum challenges conventional conceptions of learners as subordinate to the expert tutor in engaging with what is taught and how it is taught. Students are regarded as agents in the process of transformative learning (Fielding, 1999), where the aim is to strive for radical collegiality in relation to course content and approaches to learning and teaching. Co-creation within the nursing curriculum is clearly not without its challenges as it requires academic staff to be open to democratic approaches and to recognise that in certain circumstances the student will be the 'expert', having been a first-hand witness to a particular experience, which might then be shared in the classroom as a learning opportunity. Co-creation in this sense can occur at different levels, for example, students as co-creators of teaching approaches, as co-creators of course design and as co-creators of assessment strategies. All levels of co-creation significantly deepen student engagement with learning. While not without challenges, the co-created curriculum in nurse education has the potential to assist students with the transition from enacting what is required of them in order to complete the study programme (the nursing degree) and to consciously analyse what constitutes and enhances that learning, that is, what the learner knows to who the learner is (Bovill, Cook-Sather, & Felten, 2011). In the context of nurse education this is essential given the complexities of nursing practice in the current NHS, where resources are finite, staff are in short supply, and a state of uncertainly exists in terms of the political landscape and accompanying ideological assumptions regarding healthcare.

Principles of Co-creation in Education

Co-creation in education rests on the premise that creativity always resides in action. Co-creation in the curriculum requires a special form of collective action, which involves creating together with learners and teachers coming together to collectively pool insights and innovation, for the mutual benefit of the educative experience. Co-creation in education specifically involves a process in which *diverse stakeholders* are *actively* engaged in a *mutually empowering* act of *collective* creativity with *experiential* and *practical* outcomes (https://www.cocreation.world/co-creation/).

The theory of co-creation rests on the assumption that stakeholders are an integral part of the organisational team, in other words, inclusive of people on the *inside*, as opposed to invited outsiders. This is important not least because in curriculum development, practitioners often take on the role of invited *outsiders*. The role of the *outside* influence is to specifically cause creative disruption by allowing specific viewpoints and experience to reframe traditional ways of thinking. In so doing new perspectives and insights are brought to bear on the curriculum.

It is important to distinguish co-creation in education from other forms of engagement, especially where curriculum development is concerned. As is often the case a series of nested activities take place during the development process, which appear to involve collaborative action, but where positioning of the event/activity in an academic setting reinforces insider/outsider positionality. Co-creation in education should include multiple forms of collaboration, while not being defined by these. Curriculum development may involve multiple stakeholder groups, undertaking multiple activities, with nuanced co-creation manifested in what each group does within each activity, and how this contributes to the whole.

Co-creation in Nurse Education

Nurse education faces significant challenges in preparing nurses for contemporary nursing practice, for example complex issues around population demographics, increasingly complex patterns of disease, and increasing demand for and cost of technologically advanced medicine. While these challenges are experienced around the globe, inevitably low-income countries and low-income populations within countries are impacted to a greater degree than higher income countries with stable economies. Poverty, political unrest, war, and famine compound the issues by increasing the likelihood of nurses seeking to migrate to countries perceived as offering better life chances and work opportunities; the impact of which is felt exponentially in poorer countries, whose economies subsequently suffer through net migration of the nursing workforce. In responding to the challenge of educating the nursing workforce to meet these global changes, nurse academics have looked towards alternative pedagogies for nurse education. Pamela Ironside, for example, has written extensively around interpretive pedagogies, as a means of reforming nurse education for modern nursing practice (Ironside, 2006, 2014, 2015; Ironside & Hayden-Miles, 2012), concluding that while many teachers of nursing acknowledge the significance of new pedagogies, widespread use has been slow to enter mainstream nurse education, with conventional pedagogy (competency-based or outcomes education) continuing to dominate.

Alternative pedagogies for nurse education, for example, critical, feminist, postmodern and phenomenological, although different in relation to the beliefs about the nature of knowledge, provide new ways of thinking about learning and teaching, which recognise the value of the student experience to the nursing curriculum. Pedagogies such as these focus attention away from strategies covering content to strategies engendering community interpretive scholarship (Ironside, 2004). Community interpretive scholarship reflects the centrality of communal thinking directed towards interpreting encounters in practice and education from multiple perspectives (Scheckel, cited by Ironside, 2006). Community interpretive scholarship is underpinned by the principles of co-production, whereby people are considered assets, active as opposed to passive, and where relationships between participating individuals are seen as reciprocal. In education, the language most often used to describe a philosophy of co-production is co-creation.

The concept of co-creation in education is not new, generally applying to learners and teachers acting as co-constructors of knowledge. Bovill (2013) provides an explanation of the history of co-creation before concluding that while much of the literature originated in schools, there has been a recent rise in interest in a range of student partnerships in higher education. Nurse education is now firmly established in higher education, and as such nurse educators are as concerned as educators in other disciplines about student-centred learning, social learning, enquiry-based learning and learning communities. Bovill cautions however, for an avoidance of instrumental and uncritical usage of terms such as student participation, particularity in wider university strategy. Claiming participation, without offering full participation risks disengagement, with the potential for students to become disillusioned with the educational process, resulting in the perverse effect of increased attrition from nursing programmes.

A further consideration with respect to co-creation lies in the realisation that not all nurse academics and nursing students will want to be involved in co-creating the curriculum. To ignore this is to disengage from critical thinking, which recognises the process of objective analysis and evaluation before forming a judgement. In order to assess the readiness of learners and teachers to engage with co-creation, it is first necessary to consider the common understanding of 'curriculum' and 'participation'.

Curriculum is a problematic term in the sense that it is used interchangeably to refer to content, syllabus or programme of study. Definitions of curriculum have subsequently included the structure and content of a unit, the structure and content of a programme of study, the students' experience of learning or a dynamic and interactive process of teaching and learning (Fraser & Bosanquet, 2006). The former definitions focus on commonly understood ideas of curriculum, while the later tend towards broader definitions, which begin to capture the notion of shared enterprise between learning and teaching, in other words the concept of co-creation. Understanding the nature of curriculum as being more than its component parts, that is, modules, units and courses, is essential for co-creation in nurse education to work effectively. Curriculum when viewed as dynamic, emergent and collaborative allows for an expansion of conventional thinking, from one of 'teacher as expert transferring knowledge to the learner' to one of 'learner and teacher acting as co-constructors of knowledge'.

Participation, as a feature of co-creation can be as problematic a concept as curriculum, in that different ideas of participation are in evidence in education. For example, universities refer to student participation in terms of widening access, while others refer to student representation on university committees or programme boards at a variety of levels. However, as Bovill (2013) points out, there are differences between participating in university life, ensuring student voices are represented on university committees, and the idea of students becoming partners or co-creators of learning experiences. Student participation with respect to learning and teaching often takes the form of end of module, or end of programme feedback, with data usually collected via questionnaire, or at staff-student committees. Other more proactive forms of student participation might involve students as researchers, as scholars in their own learning, or as change agents in their own institutions. How student participation is conceptualised within a given curriculum depends on a collective understanding of, and readiness and willingness to embrace co-creation at institutional, departmental and individual levels.

Co-creation as previously noted, is not without its challenges. For co-creation to work in nurse education the wider political and economic context of nursing and nurse education needs to be acknowledged. First, the recent criticisms of nursing have given rise to a resurgence of calls for a refocusing on more esoteric characteristics, the enigmatic, abstract 'care and compassion', considered synonymous with nursing, but which are arguably difficult to teach in an academic setting and by implication can only be learnt in the practice setting. It necessarily follows from this argument, that nursing has no place in higher education, in which case discussions around co-creation become redundant. Second, economic instability has given rise to reassessment of funding for higher education, which has similarly impacted ways in which nurse education is financed; the full impact of which is yet to be fully evaluated. Nonetheless the marketisation of higher education in the UK, including expansion of student numbers, rising tuition fees and removal of bursaries for student nurses, makes it more difficult to argue for approaches which require ever more participation from academic staff and students.

In spite of the reservations noted above co-creation provides the means by which nurse education can achieve espoused goals to prepare nurses to meet the challenges of contemporary nursing practice. How learning and teaching is conceptualised by nurse academics will determine the degree to which co-creation is embraced within the nursing curriculum. Some approaches to co-creation are offered below.

Co-creative Approaches in the Nursing Curriculum

Nursing is conceptualised in this book as art, as science and as a personal and moral commitment. As such nursing draws on forms of nursing knowledge which support this conceptualisation: empirical, aesthetic, personal, ethical and moral. Understanding the critical dimensions of nursing requires innovative learning and teaching strategies. However, the Nursing and Midwifery Council prescribes nurse education along fairly prescriptive ways, by providing a standardised framework to which nursing programmes must adhere. While this allows for the scientific dimension of nursing to be catered for, it does not accommodate nursing as art, nor does it fully address the personal and moral commitment to nursing, which is required but not explicitly taught. The NMC (2015) describes the professional standards of practice and behaviour that all nurses and midwives registered in the UK must uphold to ensure patients, families and the public understand what can be expected from nursing and midwifery care. The challenge for nurse educators remains one of how to incorporate the esoteric, abstract 'art of nursing' into the curriculum in meaningful ways. The following section considers learning and teaching strategies, which incorporate principles of co-creation, while at the same time offering practical ideas for curriculum transformation.

Narrative Pedagogy

Narrative pedagogy is an approach to learning and teaching, a community practice and a way of thinking about what is possible and problematic in nursing (Ironside, 2003). Narrative pedagogy is manifest when students and teachers publicly share and interpret lived experiences in a mindful way, with the aim of increasing collective understanding of the experience, for the benefit of those for whom the experience is often inaccessible. The emphasis within narrative pedagogy is thus not on knowledge acquisition but more about the application of thinking to practice.

Narrative pedagogy has potential to transform conventional approaches to nurse education, which traditionally position teacher as expert and in which knowledge is considered as cognitive gain. Enacting narrative pedagogy involves conceding the idea of nursing as idealised practice, in other words revealing the hidden curriculum, dispelling a mythical romanticised version of nursing, thus allowing the true nature of contemporary nursing to be made known to the learner. By engaging in narrative pedagogy, the nurse educator mitigates the real world of nursing practice, for which students are often ill prepared, by gathering together teachers and students into converging conversations wherein many perspectives can be considered. Narrative pedagogy, in this sense, gathers together all pedagogies (Diekelmann, 2001). Learners and teachers interpret their experiences from various perspectives, including conventional, critical, feminist, postmodern and phenomenological, thus creating new possibilities for teaching thinking in classroom and clinical settings (Ironside, 2003).

Storytelling is an example of narrative pedagogy in action. As one of the oldest methods of communication, stories serve to educate others, teach cultural values, bridge generations and to share common experiences. Learning through storytelling refers to a process in which learning is structured around a narrative or story as a means of 'sense making'. Storytelling can involve the use of personal stories and/or anecdote to engage learners and to share knowledge among learners (HEA, 2017). In this sense, storytelling may include narrative approaches, case studies, life histories, myth, legend and critical incidents.

Stories are thought of as a unique way of helping students to develop respect and appreciation of other cultures and as such are directly applicable to nursing. Through stories students can explore aspects of their own culture, experience diverse cultures, empathise with the unfamiliar in terms of people/places/situations, come to understand different traditions and values and consider new ideas. With respect to nurse education, storytelling provides a vehicle through which a significant and/or treasured memory can be shared with learners for whom the experience is inaccessible or for whom the story resonates. This multidimensional aspect of storytelling permits both storyteller and listener to gain new or different perspectives on memories, thoughts and emotions, and has long been recognised as therapeutic (Chelf, Deshler, Hillman, & Durazo-Arvizu, 2000).

Storytelling in nurse education encourages active listening and develops students' skills of reflection, which are component parts of critical thinking. Conceptualising nurse education within a narrative pedagogical framework, whereby storytelling is integral to learning and teaching, not only reveals what would otherwise be hidden from the learner but enables learners to critically appraise and subsequently transfer new knowledge to other, as yet unexperienced situations. In practical terms storytelling, as a learning and teaching strategy, can be used to increase awareness of issues of relevance to nursing and nursing practice, for example, ethical dilemmas, domestic violence, inequalities in health and social injustice. Case studies, vignettes, film, text and role playing can all be used to generate stories through which emotional response, compassionate practice, reflection in and on action and critical examination of practice can be addressed (Hafford-Letchfield & Lavender, 2015). While these methods may be utilised by many nurse educators within discreet modules, units or courses, it is in only when locating storytelling within a broader pedagogical framework that coherence is achieved within the curriculum.

Storytelling, when embedded in a narrative pedagogical framework requires learners and teachers to hold a mutual understanding of co-creation in nurse education. That is to say the expectation of both teacher and student is for a curriculum underpinned by principles of mutual respect, equal participation, student and teacher as asset and active engagement in learning and teaching. In the absence of this mutual understanding and commitment to co-creation it is unlikely for the transformative potential of narrative pedagogy to be realised.

Dialogic Pedagogy

Conventional forms of nurse education are designed to maintain set values about nursing and fixed assumptions about the role of nurses in healthcare. These values and assumptions reflect the dominant groups and governing agencies in nursing; government, the public, the media, nursing's statutory body, instead of being based on democratic and political commitments to nursing. Nurse education, as a result, has been reduced to a set of pedagogical practices which emphasise a one-sided view of nursing, namely, nursing as science. This pedagogical approach, which takes a positivistic, behaviourist stance, has resulted in an 'outcomes'-based, competency-driven system of nurse education, characterised by a monological and unilateral form of pedagogy, in which the teacher imparts knowledge and the students supposedly learn it (Freire, 1972). Rather than criticise current forms of education, examination of nursing pedagogy serves to recognise the creative limitations to curriculum development, which result from rigid imposition of a regulatory framework. Nursing pedagogy should not simply be 'teaching technique' but should include all practices that define what is important to know and how it is to be known. An alternative approach to preparing nurses for modern-day nursing practice is to recognise the student's role in defining what should be learnt, in other words, dialogic pedagogy.

Dialogic pedagogy is 'critical', premised on the belief that learning takes place through egalitarian dialogue in which learners and teachers provide arguments based on a claim of validity as opposed to claims of power (Freire, 1972). In nurse education, dialogic pedagogy is transformative, enabling nursing as art, science, and a personal and moral commitment to be conveyed through dialogic teaching practices. Educators have the responsibility of identifying applicants to nurse education programmes who are compassionate or have the potential to become compassionate nurses. This is problematic because exactly what constitutes compassion is not clear, and trying to identify evidence of compassion in applicants is a difficult task. Proof that an applicant has compassion can be sought from statements on caring made on an application form, or possibly provided by a referee.

Even having selected candidates who display the necessary qualities is no guarantee that at the end of a pre-registration course, they will still have these qualities. During educational programmes, students' values may be influenced by the informal curriculum (Johnson, 2008). The informal curriculum refers to lessons that are not explicitly taught. For example, as already discussed in Chap. 5, in nursing, these might include aspects hidden within the curriculum such as activism in nursing, and the politics of nursing practice. The challenge is for the nursing curriculum to recognise the range of influences on the development of the learner and how these might be considered in relation to learning and teaching strategies. Dialogic teaching practices harness the power of talk to stimulate and extend the learners' thinking and advance learning and understanding, being as much about the teacher as the learner, and relating to teaching across the whole curriculum. A set of practices can be used to design nursing curricula to included dialogic learning and teaching. These are described below:

Dialogic Learning and Teaching in Nursing

- Knowledge is flexible, meaning different things to different people at different times.
- The needs of the learner influence learning events within the curriculum.
- The dialogue between different perspectives leads to new understandings and generates new knowledge.
- In order for learners to influence learning events, learners need to reflect on learning experiences.
- Learners need to know what they can expect of each learning event and what is expected of them.
- Learning events recognise individual learning styles and accommodate these.
- Learners and teachers are engaged in learning in an environment where differences are respected and rigorously examined.
- Learners are respected and valued. The learning environment is safe, valued and supported.
- Meanings constructed from the inside by learners in dialogue, rather than imposed from the outside, lead to powerful learning.
- Feedback and evaluation practices are dialogic, integral, communicated and acted upon.
- Learning through dialogue enhances critical thinking skills, in addition to content knowledge.

In summary, dialogic pedagogy shifts the focus to the learner and their learning, helping nursing students recognise their power as active decision-makers in their learning, which in turn helps students recognise their power as active decision-makers in nursing practice. Respect for the 'other' person's agency is central to dialogic pedagogy and fundamental to a holistic view of nursing. Dialogic teaching in nursing means using talk most effectively in learning and teaching about nursing and involves continual ongoing dialogue between learners and teachers. Through dialogue, nurse educators can elicit students' everyday common sense perspectives, engage their developing ideas and help them overcome misunderstandings. By engaging students in dialogue, teachers can explain ideas, clarify points, and help students grasp new ways of describing phenomena, including experience of practice (Alexander, 2000).

Critically Reflective Learning

Reflection in nursing has long been accepted as a necessary skill, with the definition by Boud, Keogh and Walker (1985, p19) most often used in teaching reflective practice:

> A generic term for those intellectual and affective activities in which individuals engage to explore their experiences in order to lead to new understandings and appreciations. It may take place in isolation or in association with others. It can be done well or badly, successfully or unsuccessfully.

Critical reflection is less well considered, both in nursing practice and in nurse education, although some nurse educators may use reflection and critical reflection interchangeably. For reflection to become critical its purpose needs to shift to first understand how considerations of power underpin, frame, and distort nursing and nurse education processes and interactions; and second, to unearthing and questioning the assumptions and practices that appear to make learning and teaching about nursing less problematic, but which in the longer-term work against the best interests of the profession. For example, assumptions about nursing, the role of the nurse, professional relationships, and assumptions about learning and teaching. Critically reflective teaching is a prerequisite for critically reflective learning. The addition of *critical* to *reflection* signifies a more profound consideration and focuses on the importance of:

1. Recognition and appreciation of difference and diversity within nursing and nurse education from many perspectives, for example, ethnicity, gender, culture, religion and disability
2. Challenging taken-for-granted assumptions about nursing and nurse education and the learning environment
3. Identifying and negotiating how power operates in nursing and nurse education contexts
4. Facilitating and enabling a learning and teaching environment, which challenges student nurses to think critically and morally about issues pertinent to nursing and healthcare
5. Initiating socially engaged lifelong and transformative learning

Critical reflection is central to critical pedagogy in nurse education, in that it leads students to understand how nursing practice can counteract the effects of racism, of bullying, and of other forms of structural, institutional, and organisational discrimination, which determine a nurse's ability to provide competent care, with compassion. The two-part framework below proposed by Blanchet Garneau (2016) was originally designed for cultural competence development but can equally be adapted to provide the means through which critical reflective learning becomes integral to the nursing curriculum, and is in keeping with dialogic pedagogy. Phase one is designed to pose critical questions for learners and can be used within any given area of nursing practice or theory.

Critical Reflection Process: Questions for Students (adapted with permission from Blanchet Garneau (2016))
1. What issues seem significant to pay attention to?
2. How were you feeling, and what made you feel that way?
3. What values, beliefs and assumptions guided your actions in this situation?
4. Where have these beliefs come from?

5. What social practices are expressed in these beliefs?
6. What factors constrain your views about this situation?
7. What factors may influence the way you provided care in this situation?
8. What sources of knowledge influenced or should have influenced your thinking and actions in this situation?

The second phase in Blanchet Garneau's two-phase critical reflection process invites learners to share experiences with individuals in their peer group. The teacher's role here is to facilitate dialogue and foster engagement of students in critical reflection, with the aim of validating the learners contested values, beliefs and assumptions through discourse (Blanchet Garneau, 2016, p. 133). Sharing experiences and reflection, says Blanchet Garneau, provides an opportunity for students to confront other perspectives, have assumptions and expectations challenged, and deepen and extend learning.

Blanchet Garneau suggests a thematic approach to facilitating dialogue and reflection among learners. She provides the following example:

Consideration of 'other perspectives or alternative ways of viewing the world'—for example, being able to identify what perspectives are missing from one's account.

This theme then generates questions for students to critically reflect upon, for example:

1. What were the needs of the client in this situation?
2. Were they reflecting clients' needs or organisation needs? Were you coercing the client into working with organisational needs?
3. How was the client responding?
4. What factors exist that may serve to impede the client achieving individual goals?

Critically reflective learning and teaching within the nursing curriculum is not without its challenges. Priority is usually given to fulfilling the requirements of the NMC standards for professional practice, required in order for students to be admitted to the register and thus eligible to practice. Consequently, little time remains for creativity around ways of engaging students in critically reflective activities, for example service learning, commonly referred to in the UK as student volunteering. Student volunteering is a form of experiential education in which students engage in activities that address human and community needs, together with structured opportunities designed to promote learning and development. As such, student volunteering integrates community service with academic learning. When thought of in this way student volunteering in nursing can be viewed as integral to transformative pedagogy, with potential to enable students to synthesise thoughtful reflection, caring, and action, within a theory and research-driven practice. In other words, nursing praxis is actualised through the process of student volunteering.

Critical reflection is an extension of 'critical thinking'. When used in nurse education, it asks student nurses to think about practice, and then challenges them to step back and examine that thinking by asking critical questions. For these reasons the skills of critical reflection are an imperative for nurses, in order that they may think about less than ideal situations, how these might be improved with future action and what resources might be necessary in order for improvement to take place and as such are an imperative for inclusion within the nursing curriculum. Using a critically reflective framework exposes nursing students to the 'rawness' of a critical incident before it occurs in practice, thus enabling aspects of the situation to be reflected upon in a safe environment.

Conclusion

This chapter has argued a reconsideration of nursing pedagogy is essential if nurse education is to rise to the challenge of preparing nurses for contemporary nursing practice. Population growth, complex patterns of disease, advancing technology and global migration of the nursing workforce make it necessary to conceptualise nursing as a personal and moral commitment, in addition to nursing as art and science. This holistic interpretation of nursing, informed by specific forms of knowledge, empirical, aesthetic, personal, moral and ethical, requires pedagogical approaches to nurse education, which have the capacity to transform the nursing curriculum. Pedagogies considered appropriate for transforming the nursing curriculum include narrative, dialogic and critical reflective learning. The notion of co-creation in the nursing curriculum, underpinned by principles of co-production is suggested as a means of actualising these alternative pedagogies within the curriculum.

Co-creation recognises students as assets, as active participants in learning, and acknowledges the reciprocal nature of learning and teaching in ways which enable transformational change. Transformational change results through nursing praxis, in other words when theory is embodied in practice. Structured opportunities for student volunteering are suggested as a way to provide learners with real opportunities to engage theory in action. When followed by opportunities for reflective dialogue within a safe learning environment, students are enabled to critically appraise their own values and belief systems and to critically evaluate the values and belief systems of others, of higher education institutions and of healthcare organisations. This co-created approach to curriculum design, underpinned by transformative pedagogical approaches to learning and teaching, is postulated as the way forward for nurse education and a mindful response to the recommendations of the Francis Inquiry.

The final chapter sums up key arguments for transforming nurse education through attention to alternative nursing pedagogy and subsequent curriculum development in nursing. A co-created model of nurse education is described, whereby the inclusion of structured volunteering opportunities provides the means for narrative, dialogic and critical reflective approaches to learning and teaching. In combination with a constructivist design for learning and teaching nursing competencies, the model ensures the curriculum meets the requirements of the NMC while at the same time conceptualising nursing as art, as science and as a personal and moral commitment.

References

Alexander, R. (2000). Towards dialogic teaching. Retrieved May 27, 2017, from www.robinalexander.org.uk

Blanchet Garneau, A. (2016). Critical reflection in cultural competence development: A framework for undergraduate nursing education. *Journal of Nursing Education, 55*(3), 125–132.

Boud, D., Keogh, R., & Walker, D. (1985). *Reflection: Turning experience into learning*. London: Kogan Page.

Bovill, C. (2013). Students and staff co-creating curricula: A new trend or an old idea we never got around to implementing? In C. Rust (Ed.), *Improving student learning through research and scholarship: 20 years of ISL, Improving student learning (20). Oxford Centre for Staff and Learning Development* (pp. 96–108). Oxford: OCSD.

Bovill, C., Cook-Sather, A., & Felten, P. (2011). Changing participants in pedagogical planning: Students as co-creators of teaching approaches, course design and curricula. *International Journal of Academic Development, 16*(2), 133–145.

Chelf, J. H., Deshler, A. M. B., Hillman, S., & Durazo-Arvizu, R. (2000). Storytelling: A strategy for coping with cancer. *Cancer Nursing, 23*(1), 1–5.

Diekelmann, N. (2001). Narrative pedagogy: Heideggerian hermeneutical analyses of lived experiences of students, teachers, and clinicians. *Advances in Nursing Science, 23*(3), 53–71.

Fielding, M. (1999). Radical collegiality: Affirming teaching as an inclusive professional practice. *Australian Educational Researcher, 26*(2), 1–34.

Fraser, S., & Bosanquet, A. (2006). The curriculum? That's just a unit outline, isn't it? *Studies in Higher Education, 31*(3), 269–284.

Freire, P. (1972). *Pedagogy of the oppressed*. London: Penguin Books.

Hafford-Letchfield, T., & Lavender, P. (2015). Quality improvement through the paradigm of learning. *Quality in Ageing and Older Adults, 16*(4), 1–13.

Higher Education Academy. (2017). Learning through storytelling. Retrieved May 28, 2017, from https://www.heacademy.ac.uk/enhancement/starter-tools/learning-through-storytelling

Ironside, P. M. (2003). New pedagogies for teaching thinking: The lived experiences of students and teachers enacting narrative pedagogy. *Journal of Nursing Education, 42*, 509–516.

Ironside, P. M. (2004). "Covering content" and teaching thinking: Deconstructing the additive curriculum. *Journal of Nursing Education, 43*(1), 5–12.

Ironside, P. M. (2006). Using narrative pedagogy: Learning and practising interpretive thinking. *Journal of Advanced Nursing, 55*(4), 478–486.

Ironside, P. M. (2014). Enabling narrative pedagogy: Inviting, waiting and letting-be. *Nursing Education Perspectives, 35*(3), 212–218.

Ironside, P. M. (2015). Narrative pedagogy: Transforming nursing education through of research. *Nursing Education Perspectives, 36*(2), 83–88.

Ironside, P. M., & Hayden-Miles, M. (2012). Narrative pedagogy: Co-creating engaging learning experiences with students. In G. Sherwood & S. Horton-Deutsch (Eds.), *Reflective practice: Transforming education and improving outcomes* (pp. 135–148). Indianapolis, IN: Sigma Theta Tau International.

NMC. (2015). *The code: Professional standards of practice and behaviour for nurses and midwives.* NMC, London. Retrieved from www.nmc-uk.org

7

Preparing Nurses for Contemporary Nursing Practice

Introduction

Nursing and nurse education are inextricably linked; criticism of one necessarily implies criticism of the other. The NMC, in part as a response to concerns around nursing and nurse education identified within the Francis Report, called for a consultation on arrangements for the revalidation process for nurses and midwives seeking to remain on the professional register. Prior to the new arrangements, the NMC had no power to seek information from a third party to verify claims of competency made by practising nurses and midwives. However, under the new arrangements, which came into force from April 2016, an enhanced system of appraisal sees nurses and midwives having to reflect on the views of patients, users and colleagues in order to demonstrate continued ability to practise safely and effectively. Revalidation places the onus on nurses and midwives to demonstrate, through practice related feedback, written reflective accounts and reflective discussion, that they have met the requirements. In addition, nurses and midwives are asked to confirm they are of good health and good character, which essentially requires disclosure of criminal offences or formal cautions, as well as declaring appropriate professional indemnity is in place. Once all requirements are met, an appropriate person or 'confirmer' looks at the evidence and confirms, in a process repeated every 3 years, that all revalidation requirements have been met (NMC, 2016b). While the NMC hopes this rigorous approach to revalidation will strengthen public confidence in the nursing and midwifery profession, the new arrangements have been subject to criticism, not least by the Royal College of Nursing through a survey of its members.

The RCN's independent survey highlighted members concerns around the principle and practicalities of the revalidation process, including whether appraisal is in fact a legitimate feature of revalidation, and whether the NMC had the infrastructure to support the process. According to RCN members the purpose of appraisal (for employers to review performance in a given role) and of revalidation (to confirm fitness to remain on the NMC register) are entirely separate. Moreover, conflating the two poses a significant risk of confusion and unacceptable outcomes (RCN, 2014). Concern was also expressed over the failure of the NMC to make a clear separation between its employment and regulatory functions, reminiscent of concerns previously raised by the Council for Healthcare Regulatory Excellence, who found the NMC had not understood its regulatory functions well (CHRE, 2012). Notwithstanding the validity of the concerns raised, revalidation is clearly designed to protect patient safety and to support a culture of professionalism, and in this respect the NMC has taken important steps. To this end nurse education needs to work alongside the NMC to design nursing programmes, which can guarantee public trust and confidence in the graduate nurse. With this in mind this concluding chapter considers what nurse educators can do to design and deliver a nursing curriculum fit for the purpose of preparing nurses for contemporary nursing practice. The chapter begins by revisiting factors impacting nurse education, as a prerequisite for exploration of approaches to curriculum development in nursing.

Contextual Issues Impacting Nurse Education

The public inquiry into failings at Mid Staffordshire NHS Foundation Trust clearly signified the arrival of a new era, not just for healthcare and for nursing, but also for nurse education. While the Royal College of Nursing and the Nursing and Midwifery Council supported nurses in the aftermath of the Francis Inquiry, nevertheless the inquiry provided the public, the media and politicians with an opportunity to refocus attention on how and where nurses are educated. Nurses, so the argument goes, do not need a degree in order to learn how to care, and therefore nurse 'training' has no place in higher education, being something which can be taught and learnt in clinical settings. Arguments such as these lead to the strongly contested assertion that returning to apprenticeship type training affords a solution to the concerns around the calibre of nurses, including students. The spurious notion that the training of nurses as opposed to the education of nurses provides remedy for an ailing health and social care system diverts attention away from pedagogical solutions of real value to nurses, nurse students and nursing. On the contrary, nurse education should remain situated within higher education in order for nurse educators to displace reactionary pedagogies, which oppose political and/or social progress in nursing, in favour of progressive pedagogies, which emphasise problem solving, critical thinking, and which are firmly rooted in present nursing experience. Nursing students deserve the best possible educational experience; one where they can learn along with and alongside students from many other disciplines. While there is a valid argument that students accrue high levels of debt from studying at university, with this set to worsen with replacement of the student bursary with loan arrangement, nevertheless a university education produces tangible benefits for nursing students. University education exposes students to new research and technologies, encourages independent thought and creativity, offers the chance for new experiences, including overseas travel, and exposes students to other cultures and backgrounds (Furnham, 2014). More to the point though, a university education for nursing students was a long time coming, hard won and should not be relinquished, at least not without sound evidence that reverting to hospital-based training produces nurses who are better able to care, more compassionate, more professional and more deserving of public trust. The negativity, which often characterises reporting about nursing, is counteracted by the national summary of results of the 2012 Inpatients Survey, whereby 80% of respondents reported that overall they were always treated with respect and dignity while they were in hospital. Despite the negative image of nurses, it would seem the general public do have confidence in the profession (McSherry, 2013). The challenge for nurse educators is to develop appropriate pedagogies for nursing, while taking account of the current context of uncertainty around health and social care.

Health and Social Care: Educating for Uncertainty

Major changes in healthcare systems and the environments in which nurses practice require profound changes to the way in which nurses are educated. Demographic changes, changing patterns of disease, increasing levels of acute and chronic disability in the short and medium term, impact the way in which services are delivered, and subsequently impact conceptualisation of nurse education. A key function of nurse education therefore has to be to provide nurses with the requisite skills for continual adaptation to the uncertain health and social care environments, which characterise contemporary nursing practice.

People are living longer. The population of England has increased from 41 million in 1951 to 53 million in 2012, with the longer-term projection suggesting the population is set to reach 61 million by 2032 (Ham, Dixon, & Brooke, 2012). These population increases are accompanied by a rise in people over age 65, with a subsequent change in the balance between people in this age group and those of working age (Ham et al., 2012). Increases in 'older old', that is, people over age 85, are particularly important in relation to health and social care services, in that increased longevity is inevitably accompanied by increased demand for and use of health and social care services. While people living longer is a cause for celebration and as Britnell (2015) suggests is in part testament in the UK to the NHS, which is still considered the proudest achievement of modern society, nevertheless increases in life expectancy are not necessarily associated with lives lived in better health. Understanding the relationship between health, healthcare services and nursing is fundamental for nurse education if it is to be successful in preparing nurses for modern nursing practice.

Advancing Technology and Changing Expectations

Advances in medical care, including drugs, surgical procedures and diagnostic procedures have contributed to improvements in population health and outcomes of care (Ham et al., 2012). The Human Genome

Project, completed in 2003, has successfully mapped the sequence of the human genome, which is thought to enable medical science to develop highly effective diagnostic tools, to better understand the health needs of people based on their individual genetic make-up and to design new and highly effective treatments for disease. Mapping the human genome has thus signalled a new age of discovery for the transformation of human health. This proliferation of knowledge creates a challenge for health professionals to keep up to date with the evidence base for conditions and subsequent treatments, which were previously unavailable. However, this 'explosion' of knowledge is not confined to healthcare professionals, being readily available to patients, families and carers, thus having the potential to change the nature of the relationship of patients and professionals, one with the other.

The implications of advancing technology, changing expectations and changing professional relationships impact nurse education, in that the nursing curriculum needs to be responsive to changes to how and where nursing is practised and by whom. The primary goal of nurse education must remain one of preparing nurses to meet the diverse needs of patients, their families and their carers, while at the same time paying attention to the need for nurses to act as agents of change, to be leaders within nursing, and to be at the forefront of decisions made about the direction of nursing, as a profession and as an academic discipline. How successful the nursing curriculum is in meeting the aims and objectives of nurse education is determined by how well nurse educators are able to draw on theories and practice in curriculum development.

The Role of Nurse Educators in Curriculum Development

Nurse educators have the dual role of educators and nurses. However, while a nursing qualification implies the requirements of a pre-registration programme have been met with subsequent admission to the NMC register, the nurse educator role is often driven by the need for teaching in a specific area (palliative care, intensive care, emergency care, paediatrics), and not necessarily by educational expertise. A Postgraduate Certificate in Higher Education (PGCHE) or equivalent is often a secondary factor in the appointment of a nurse lecturer with the practitioner's level of clinical acumen being of prime importance. The requirement to undertake a PGCHE, usually within 1 year of appointment, is often a condition of service, as opposed to a condition of appointment. Course content and learning outcomes within PGCHE programmes may vary considerably, although alignment with the Higher Education Academy's UK Professional Standards Framework (UKPSF) does provide a degree of consistency. Nurse lecturers, new to teaching in a university may opt to undertake the additional NMC Recordable Teacher Qualification (NMC RTQ), which enables a teaching qualification to be recorded upon completion of the necessary competencies. The NMC RTQ focuses on the pragmatics of teaching and learning, as opposed to content around theories underpinning curriculum development, which invariably means a nurse educator may be a competent teacher without having the necessary knowledge required for curriculum development. Nevertheless, nurse educators should be prepared to explore the theoretical assumptions underpinning a given nursing curriculum and take measures to ensure such knowledge underpins their educational practice, whether through formal mechanisms (postgraduate studies in learning and teaching) or through independent study.

Theories and Practice in Curriculum Development

In general terms, curriculum broadly refers to all *planned* learning. In this sense curriculum encompasses the totality of a learners' experiences, occurring as a result of the educational process (Kelly, 2009). Two features are worthy of note within this notion of curriculum. First, that learning is planned and guided and occurs in groups or individually, and second, that curriculum theory and practice is rooted in the notion of *place*, which may be inside or outside formal settings. There are a number of ways to envisage curriculum theory and practice, namely, curriculum as a body of knowledge, as an attempt to achieve certain ends in students (a product) and as a process in and of itself, or curriculum as praxis, that is, as theory enacted. In general, the approach to curriculum theory and practice determines the dominant model for curriculum design, bearing in mind the context in which a given curriculum operates. The nursing curriculum in the UK is specifically determined by its regulatory body (the NMC), who demand a set of educational standards and require evidence of exposure to specified periods of education in theory and practice settings. In this sense, the approach to curriculum theory and practice in nursing is predetermined to a large extent. Nevertheless, it is the responsibility of nurse educators to bring to bear a sound knowledge of educational theory when undertaking curriculum development in nursing.

Curriculum Models

Defining an appropriate curriculum model is the first step in curriculum development, with the choice of model ultimately determining the type of curriculum produced. The curriculum model encompasses the collective belief about the purpose and point of education, and the approach and subsequent methods for learning and teaching. The point and purpose for education is manifest in the curriculum model in a number of ways: *focus*, which looks at a subject or student and centres instruction on them; *approach*, which looks at the type of instruction to be used; *content*, which looks at the topic or subject and how these will be written within the curriculum; *process*, which looks at assessment, that is, formative and summative; and *structure*, which looks at how the curriculum will be evaluated or reviewed (Ravi, 2016).

Curriculum as Product or Process

Product curriculum models are premised on the belief that the curriculum itself leads to some kind of desirable end product, for example knowledge of certain facts, mastery over certain skills and competencies, and acquisition of certain attitudes and behaviours (Sheehan, 1986).

The best-known model of this type is that developed by Tyler in the 1940s, which uses a simple four-step approach to the curriculum. John (2006) describes the steps in the Tyler model as first, determine what students need to do in order to be successful. Each subject is considered to have natural objectives, which indicate mastery, and all objectives need to be consistent with the philosophy of the school. Step two involves developing learning experiences, which help the students to achieve the first step. Step three relates to the organisation of the experiences, for example, the approach taken towards learning and teaching, that is, should teaching come first followed by learning or vice versa. The preference is determined by the philosophy of the teacher and the perceived needs of the learners. While either sequence is thought to work, the teacher needs to adopt a logical order of experiences for learners. Step four requires the teacher to assess whether learning has taken place, through an evaluation of the learning objectives. Behavioural objectives provide the foundations on which product curriculum models are built, with the intended outcome (the product) of a learning experience prescribed beforehand. However, setting behavioural objectives at the outset can be problematic in that educational outcomes are often unpredictable and therefore hard to specify (Sheehan, 1986).

Process curriculum models in contrast to product models take a more open-ended approach. The emphasis in process models is placed on continuous development, with outcomes perceived in terms of how thinking, feeling and attitudes are developed within the learner. Process models conceptualise the curriculum as a process involving interactions between teachers, learners and knowledge, as opposed to a physical entity embodied within a set of curriculum documents. Curriculum as process asks teachers to think critically in action, to understand their role and the expectations others have of them, and to propose actions which set out the essential features of the educational encounter (Smith, 2000). Process models require teachers to encourage conversations between, and with, people in the situation, out of which may come thinking and action, and to continually evaluate the process. The curriculum thus develops through the dynamic interaction of action and reflection.

The choice of curriculum model, be it product or process depends on an understanding of what each model has to offer with respect to how education is conceptualised. However, as Sheehan (1986) points out the ultimate choice of curriculum model may have as much to do with the chooser as with anything else. Where the dominant voice emphasises the importance of predetermined behavioural objectives, it is likely that a product curriculum model will ensue. Product models also lend themselves to measurement, where such measurability implies accountability. As such product models are able to provide evidence of whether or not objectives have been met and this is clearly important to some education providers. On the other hand, process models are seen as less dehumanising, and this in itself lends process models more readily to situations where learning is seen as an active process, and where the emphasis in education is placed on independent and individualised learning. It is entirely possible to combine the best features of product and process models, should there be sound educational reasons for doing so.

Curriculum Models for Nursing: The Nursing Curriculum as a Body of Knowledge

Historic accounts of nurse training in the UK are held within the National Archives, Kew. These historic documents describe a training syllabus for the Certificate of General Nursing, whereby a concise statement of intent enabled the derivation of a series of subjects, which then made areas for examination possible. A syllabus approach to curriculum theory and practice in nursing is underpinned by the philosophical assumption that curriculum is a body of nursing knowledge with distinguishable content and/or subjects. Education, in this sense, is the process by which these are transmitted or delivered to students by the most effective methods that can be devised (Smith, 2000). Where the curriculum equates with the notion of a syllabus albeit in this simplistic fashion, then curriculum planning is concerned to a great extent with how the body of knowledge is transmitted, in other words the focus tends towards strategies for learning and teaching, rather than more complex theoretical considerations.

The Nursing Curriculum as Product

The dominant mode of describing and indeed of managing current approaches to the nursing curriculum conforms to notions of curriculum as product (Smith, 2000). In this form, nurse education is characterised by a pre-formed plan and set of objectives, leading to measurable outcomes (products). This technical rational model facilitates a particular discourse, whereby the purpose of the nursing curriculum is to *produce* nurses who are described as 'fit for purpose, award, and practice' (Benton, 2011). Discourse such as this in nurse education allows for external forces to impact curriculum development to the detriment of more appropriate forms of pedagogies for nursing. Curriculum as product is less concerned with how to articulate a vision for nursing and nurse education and more concentred with what its objectives and content might be.

The obvious attraction in viewing the nursing curriculum as product lies with its attention to describing what nurses need to know in order to function in contemporary nursing practice. Theorising the curriculum as product inevitably sees nursing programmes broken into elements, with lists of competencies identified within each component part. The resultant curriculum is reminiscent of earlier training programmes, albeit located within the academic setting, which may account for nurse education's perennial difficulty to articulate a rationale for its continued presence within HE, and the resurging view of nurses as 'too clever to care' and 'too posh to wash' (Scott, 2004). Theorising the nursing curriculum as product raises concerns around the absence of a social vision to guide the process of curriculum construction. In other words, curriculum as product inevitably directs attention towards the immediate concern to supply nursing labour for the workforce, whereas nursing curriculum when viewed as *process* places emphasis on the interaction of teachers, students and knowledge, in what happens in the theory and practice settings and on what nurse educators actually do to design, deliver and evaluate the efficacy of nurse education.

The Nursing Curriculum as Process

The nursing curriculum, when viewed as *process* takes account of two important factors in nurse education. First is the context in which learning and teaching about nursing takes place, and second, the teacher (nurse educator) enters the educational setting (classroom or practice) with a considered idea of the purpose of the encounter. In this sense, the purpose of the nursing curriculum is to communicate the essential principles and features of nursing in order for it to be open to scrutiny and capable of effective translation into practice. The idea of curriculum as process is drawn from the work of Stenhouse (1975), who argued for a curriculum grounded in practice, but one which is subject to experiment. In nurse education, this is taken to mean a curriculum, which is effectively communicated to and communicated on by teachers and by others, and raises the question of who should be involved in curriculum development. The legitimate question of stakeholder involvement in curriculum development raises a broader question of how the curriculum, when viewed as *process*, differs from education. In articulating the difference, Stenhouse took curriculum to mean the basis for planning, studying and justifying a course. In this sense, the nursing curriculum should articulate the intention of nurse education through the deliberate actions of nurse educators, which goes some way towards determining who should and should not be involved in curriculum development.

A number of steps are important when adopting a *process* approach to the nursing curriculum, which include as minimum planning the programme, studying the programme and justifying the programme:

1. Planning—what is to be learnt or taught, how is it to be learnt or taught, in what sequence will it be learnt or taught, and what differentiation might be needed between students in order for learning and teaching to be effective, that is, how will learners with different learning needs be accommodated in order to maximise potential.
2. Empirical Study (content)—what principles will be used to evaluate learning and teaching (assessment of learning, evaluation of teaching), what is the feasibility for delivering learning and teaching in different

settings/environments/contexts (NHS, social care setting, voluntary sector organisations, university), and what are the effects of different settings for learning and teaching on learners and teachers and how will these be evaluated (methods for information gathering, feedback, communication).
3. Justification—how will the intention of the nursing curriculum be made available for public scrutiny, who can access the curriculum (learners, teachers, the public, professional bodies), what mechanisms of communication or modes of access will be employed (intranet, social media, restricted/unrestricted).

Nurse education, embodied within the nursing curriculum, whereby curriculum is considered as *process* moves away from the notion of curriculum as simply a *syllabus* or body of knowledge to be conveyed to learners. Rather nurse education becomes translatable to nursing practice, open to evaluation and critical scrutiny. Nursing curricula in this sense are able to exhibit unique features, which invite rather than simply accept regulatory requirements for entry onto the professional register. A process approach to curriculum theory and practice, instead of specifying behavioural objectives and methods in advance, recognises the need for students and teachers to work together to develop content (Stenhouse, 1975), thus opening up opportunities for a co-creation in the nursing curriculum. Student nurses are not objects to be acted upon as with a product model whereby a pre-specified plan directs learning and teaching. A process model makes learning the central endeavour of teachers, with the educational setting the place where students make sense of learning about nursing (Grundy, 1987).

The Nursing Curriculum as Praxis

Nurse educators (teachers) generally enter nurse education after some considerable time in the practice setting, but with a variety of reasons for doing so. Most will have a shared commitment to delivering nurse education to the highest standard, while also having the ability to think critically about nursing practice. Embedded within the role and expectations of the nurse educator is the requirement for an understanding of theory and practice in curriculum development, and it is this which may be less well developed for nurse educators whose clinical expertise determined appointment to the role. Knowledge of theories and practice in curriculum development are important however, in that educational theories permit ways of thinking about nurse education and nursing, which facilitate the shift in thinking required for the nursing curriculum to be understood as *praxis*. Praxis is concerned with how theory is enacted, embodied or realised (Freire, 1972). Praxis in the nursing curriculum encourages nurse educators to continually engage with others through interaction and reflection to evaluate the process, in order for the curriculum to remain dynamic. In this way, the nursing curriculum is implemented through an active process, whereby the programme is planned, delivered and evaluated in an integrated fashion, in other words reciprocally related, rather than simple delivery of programme plans (Grundy, 1987).

The nursing curriculum as praxis acknowledges the collective understandings and practices of all those involved in the delivery of nurse education, thus recognising the equal partnership of nurse educators and nurse practitioners. Meaningful recognition, as opposed to simply inviting practice partners to participate in curriculum development is central to a nursing curriculum, which embodies praxis. Curriculum as praxis moves beyond exclusive focus on individuals towards a more fuller understanding of the collective experience of the people involved in nursing work, for example an understanding of the conditions in which nurses' work and which inform contemporary attitudes about nursing. The nursing curriculum as praxis has potential to reveal those otherwise hidden issues, such as working conditions, politics of nursing, inequalities and injustices in health and social care. Praxis thus requires commitment to reflection on what learning is taking place, the optimal place for learning, on teaching, and on what is being taught.

In addition to the general discussion around curriculum models, it should be noted that there are models associated with specific topics, for example, cultural awareness and cultural competence, clinical competency and public health, which have not been considered here. Cultural diversity is an issue of concern to all nurses and indeed to all health workers. As such the nursing curriculum should provide a foundation for the development of cultural competence that allows for the acquisition of the knowledge, skills and attitudes required of nurses working in diverse cultural settings (Reyes, Hadley, & Davenport, 2013). In terms of models for teaching cultural competency in nursing, choice is very much dependent on whether cultural competence is seen as a process, an outcome, or a skill which enables nurses to embrace diversity (Rumay Alexander, 2008). Irrespective of which model is ultimately chosen, engaging nurses in deliberate learning, such as is required for cultural competency requires reflection, critical reflection and active learning, and in this sense fits well with principles of co-creation.

Approaches to teaching clinical competency include a model of Situated Learning in Nursing Leadership, which is based on the work of Lave and Wenger (1991) and Benner et al's (2009) description of situated learning. The model guides the education of nursing students in leadership with consideration for the need for socialisation and practice in leadership. Learning about leadership is combined with opportunities to practice it in context, and to acquire the reasoning to move from individual patient care concerns to group/population concerns and system solutions, and then from awareness to clinical leadership (Ailey, Lamb, Friese, & Christopher, 2015). With respect to teaching about public health, there are specific approaches and/or models, although these are usually concerned with the education of specialist community practitioners (health visitors). Nevertheless, it is noted here that specialist areas of nursing deserve close attention within the undergraduate nursing curriculum and in terms of specific approaches to learning and teaching should not simply be treated as components parts of the curriculum without due consideration of appropriate learning and teaching strategies.

The Nursing Curriculum in Context

Competency-based education in nursing has long been valued and will continue to be so. The need to ensure nurses are competent is rightly seen as the corner stone of NMC approaches to standards for pre-registration education. Competency in nursing relates not only to fundamental nursing care but also to higher level competencies, for example, mastery over care management, highly complex and technical skills, decision-making and leadership across a wide range of care settings and clinical environments. In order to ensure nurses can demonstrate the full range of competencies, the curriculum has tended towards an essentially positivist, behaviour-focused, outcomes-driven framework, with the result that nurse education has focused on what nurses necessarily 'do' as opposed to how nurses 'think' (Ironside, 2004).

Despite the NMC's concern to strengthen public confidence in the nursing and midwifery profession, nurses are criticised for a lack of behaviour synonymous with nursing, that is, caring and compassionate practice. Benner et al. (2009) suggest while students appear to graduate with ample factual knowledge of core competencies they often do not appear to have a sense of how competencies can be applied or integrated into the real world of practice. Consideration needs to be given to alternative pedagogies for nursing, and a rethinking of nursing curricula to enable nurses to be properly prepared for practice.

Rethinking Nursing Pedagogy

Transforming nurse education through examination of alternative pedagogy is receiving much attention. Pamela Ironside in the USA has written extensively around pedagogy in nursing, in particular, narrative pedagogy. She argues narrative pedagogy helps students to challenge their assumptions and think through and interpret situations they encounter from multiple perspectives (Ironside, 2006). Narrative pedagogy is of importance in nursing education, since its key role is not only to ensure nurses are competent practitioners, but also to provide them with the skills to challenge assumptions, particularly in difficult situations, where patients, families and carers raise concerns about care. Narrative pedagogy does this by enabling students to share accounts of poor practice with teachers in a safe environment. By pooling wisdom students are able to challenge preconceptions, and envision different possibilities for engaging with others to ensure patient-centred care and safety. Furthermore, by using narrative pedagogy in nursing courses, teachers are encouraged to shift attention from an epistemological focus, and from strategies aimed at covering content to one which engenders community scholarship (Ironside, 2006).

Margaret McAllister, an Australian academic cautions nurse teachers to be aware of dominate modes of teaching, which can be silencing and disempowering. She explores how transformative learning supports teachers to awaken students to issues that demand all our attention. Activities within the curriculum, she argues, need to be purposeful so they activate learners to generate solutions to world problems, of relevance to practice (McAllister, 2010). A further example of the use of transformative pedagogy in nursing is provided by the Canadian scholar Amélie Blanchet Garneau who describes a critical anti-discriminatory pedagogy for nursing. She argues while nursing has a unique contribution to advancing social justice in healthcare practices and education, and although social justice has been claimed as a core value of nursing, there is little guidance regarding how to enact social justice in nursing practice and education. Blanchet Garneau and colleagues propose a critical anti-discriminatory pedagogy (CAPD) for nursing, which is grounded in a critical intersectional perspective of discrimination and which aims to foster transformative learning involving a praxis-oriented critical consciousness (Blanchet Garneau, Browne, & Varcoe, 2016).

The theoretical argument for using transformative pedagogy in nursing has been made in this book, with examples given of notable scholars responsible over time for developing transformative theories of adult learning (Mezirow) and critical pedagogy (Freire, Giroux), The following section considers how volunteering, when offered as a structured activity within the curriculum acts as a transformative pedagogy, provides students and teachers with opportunities for critical reflection, and provides a vehicle for nurse academics to engage in dialogic learning and teaching methods. In this sense, volunteering is integral to pedagogy, rather than an activity within pedagogy.

Volunteering as Pedagogy

The particular benefits of volunteering to nursing students centre on increasing the variety of social groups or situations to which students are exposed, increasing self-confidence; breaking down hierarchies, greater reflection on their own practice through doing (praxis), the development of more critical perspectives and improvements in terms of meeting particular competencies (Bell, Tanner, Rutty, Astley-Pepper, & Hall, 2014). The development of praxis and critical perspectives as part of nurse education may be one way in which progress towards greater compassion in nursing practice may be achieved, although research is needed to fully appreciate the process by which this is achieved. Nevertheless, the absence of volunteering in nursing pedagogy is a missed opportunity to harness the students' knowledge and skills; pre-existing and underpinned by the nursing programme, for the benefit of recipients of health and social care services. While student volunteering may not automatically result in learning, nor link directly to the development of caring and compassionate practice, nonetheless volunteering does provide a way for students to make sense of their experiences through opportunities intentionally designed to foster critical thinking (Dyson, Liu, van den Akker, & O'Driscoll, 2017).

Building structured opportunities for student volunteering within the curriculum may prove problematic for reasons that nursing students, on a full-time course often have to work to supplement their income, and may have additional caring or family responsibilities. In these circumstances, volunteering may be an unrealistic use of time. However, structured volunteering, when supported within the framework of the curriculum does have potential to contribute to both the achievement of competencies and the acquisition of the more esoteric and abstract qualities associated with nursing. A structured volunteering activity, followed with students' reflection on the volunteering experience provides the vehicle by which nursing praxis can be achieved. When students are encouraged to reflect on a volunteering experience they are less likely to engage in hierarchical thinking and more likely to adopt a critical stance towards health and healthcare practice, which positions the patient, client, families and carers as central to the endeavour, as opposed to the needs of the organisation. Reflection on a volunteering activity is likely to lead students to develop a more holistic view of society which acknowledges the importance of inequality and power relationships in understanding the needs of patients. Volunteering gives students the opportunity to be part of a critical pedagogy, enabling them to gain life experiences and have a sense of control over their learning, which is not always possible through traditional teaching (Bell et al., 2014).

A contentious issue, however, concerns whether or not the structured volunteering activities should be located within a discreet module, which might then be subject to assessment. Should this be the approach taken then reflective writing provides one way in which students might accrue university credits. Bell et al. (2014) describe a volunteering module, which attracts university credits. Students taking the module are required to undertake 100 hours of volunteering placements and complete an academic assignment. The module provides volunteering opportunities, which allow students to work with other partner organisations in the locality and which can be spread across the 3-year programme. In similar fashion, Hafford-Letchfield, Thomas and McDonald (2016) describe a 'community project' module, within a Bachelor of Social Work programme. The community project module is designed to enhance social work students' theoretical understanding of the context and background factors influencing the nature of social problems and society's responses. Within the module, learning and teaching strategies enable students to engage with critical theories (Freire, Habermas, Foucault) of community, sustainability, citizenship and participation through examination of critical sociology and social policy and the institutions and structures that support service users and carers at a local level. The module provides students with opportunities to prepare for professional practice and to develop a range of direct skills such as active enquiry, synthesis and evaluation of information about the socio-economic and political realities in their local community. Through selected project work students are able to make direct contact with the public and organisations providing support in their local community, and it is this aspect of the module which provides the basis for reflective analysis, which then assists students to produce a portfolio of evidence to demonstrate the integration of theory with practice. The module accrues 30 credits and includes a minimum of 5 days' voluntary work.

Access to volunteering opportunities is key to influencing choice to volunteer (McBride & Lough, 2010). While there are ways other than via the curriculum, through which nursing students are able to access volunteering opportunities, for example, through the activities of student unions, by accessing information on university websites and through attendance at induction events or 'fresher's week', an unmotivated student is unlikely to take up volunteering, particularly when studies are seen as a priority and where the demands of a programme are such that students cannot commit the necessary time (Dyson et al., 2017). Motivation to volunteer has been linked to previous volunteering experience, ready access to information, the availability of formal volunteering programmes, and support for volunteering (Jones & Hill, 2003. In the absence of access to information and support, it is unlikely students, in particular those on undergraduate nursing programmes will engage with volunteering, and as such will miss an opportunity to appreciate how volunteering impacts learning about nursing.

In summary, while volunteering is considered a mutually beneficial relationship or exchange, with considerable evidence of health and well-being benefits to those who volunteer (Morrow-Howell, 2010; Mundle, Naylor, & Buck, 2012; Paylor, 2011), measuring these benefits is complex. Meaningful evaluation of the benefits of volunteering calls for sophisticated and rigorous research designs, which are not always possible. Thus, any generalisations made from research around volunteering must be very cautious as most of the studies have limitations, which make establishing causal relationships or even strong associations between good health and well-being outcomes and volunteering difficult (Mundle et al., 2012). While there is considerable evidence of benefits to those who receive help from volunteers and to the organisations that use volunteers, such benefits are hard to evaluate and are highly dependent on context, such as the nature of the volunteering, the match between the volunteer and the person receiving help or the training received by the volunteer. Providing structured volunteering opportunities within the nursing curriculum is one way in which students might be offered an opportunity to undergo a meaning perspective transformation. The volunteering experience may cause a significant level of disruption or disturbance for the student, and in that respect, can be likened to Mezirow's description of a disorientating dilemma. Disorientating dilemmas, previously discussed in Chap. 4, can be quite modest, for example a new experience such as a volunteering activity, which prompts the student to become disorientated and thus to examine and reflect on life prior to the experience. The volunteering activity acts as a disorientating dilemma, which then facilitates critical reflection, whereby the student is assisted by the teacher to examine previously held values, attitudes, beliefs and underlying tacit assumptions, but within the safe environment of the classroom. It is important to note within this model that critical reflection cannot occur without the student first experiencing a disorientating dilemma. A structured approach to critical reflection, whereby the teacher guides the student through the process facilitates a shift in meaning perspective.

Critical Reflection on Volunteering

The following framework, adapted with permission from Renigere (2014) can be used to assist nurse teachers to optimise the process of critical reflection by ensuring the essential elements (content, process and premise) are considered within a given set of reflective activities (Mezirow, 1991). Table 7.1 depicts how the teacher guides the process of reflection on a volunteering activity undertaken by the student, using appropriate pedagogies to support reflective activities, for example, dialogic pedagogy, narrative pedagogy, storytelling, case studies, vignettes, film, text and role playing (see Chap. 6 for full explanation). The reflective process may take place during one-to-one supervision, in small group tutorials, in the practice or educational setting, and will be determined by the

Table 7.1 Facilitated reflection on a volunteering activity

   1. **Reflection on content**—what happened?
   Corresponding Reflective Activity
      - Please describe the volunteering experience is as much detail as possible
   2. **Reflection on process**—what did the volunteering experience mean to you?
   Corresponding Reflective Activity
      - Please describe any particular issues, concerns, activities, strategies and/or decisions made by the volunteer and recipient
   3. **Reflection on premise/underlying assumptions**—what do you think was happening?
   Corresponding Reflective Activity
      - Please describe what you think influenced what happened/was happening

educational philosophy underpinning curriculum design, the approach taken to adult learning, and the resources available to the curriculum, including time and availability of teaching staff. A series of nested questions can be used to prompt the reflective process.

Increasing the level of complexity of reflection on the volunteering activity leads to a shift in the student's meaning perspective. By moving beyond a simple description of events student and teacher are able, through rational discourse, to arrive at a deeper level of understanding of the event. This deeper level of reflection may involve examination of the social, political, environmental and economic factors impacting the experience of the volunteer and the recipient of the volunteering activity (Table 7.2).

The reflective questions within the framework described here are not exhaustive, and many nurse educators will already be using a variety of methods for engaging students in reflection in and on theory and practice in nursing. However, the framework is unique in that it brings together a number of constructs. First, providing a structured volunteering activity within the curriculum enables students to experience a *disorientating dilemma*, or one which acts as a catalyst for perspective transformation. Second, structuring reflection around a disorientating dilemma provides an opportunity for student and teacher to engage with a variety of critical pedagogies as part of the reflective process, for example, dialogic, narrative, storytelling, media and the arts. Third, rational discourse between learner and teacher is predicated on co-creation within the curriculum; in other words, the student is valued as an equal partner in learning and teaching about nursing.

The final section of this book proposes a co-created curriculum model for nursing. The co-created model embodies the key messages articulated thus far, namely the need to ensure decisions made around curriculum development are underpinned by a sound of knowledge of theories and practice in curriculum development, including theories of adult learning, and by consideration of transformative pedagogies for learning and teaching about nursing. Nursing, in this co-created model is conceptualised within this model as art, as science, and as a personal and moral commitment. Providing opportunities for students to volunteer is the route through which co-creation occurs within the model, in that students and

Table 7.2 Levels of reflection on a volunteering activity

1. **Emotional reflection**—understanding how one feels regarding perception, thoughts behaviours, attitudes

Corresponding Reflective Activity
- How did you *feel* about the volunteering activity? How useful do you feel it has been to you and to others involved in the volunteering activity? What in particular do you feel was most beneficial for you as the volunteer and for others involved, and why?

2. **Evaluative reflection**—evaluation of the effectiveness of the perception, thoughts behaviours, attitudes

Corresponding Reflective Activity
- What *evidence* is available to assist/develop your understanding of the volunteering experience (discussion around appropriate/relevant theories; nursing and/or other academic disciplines as necessary)

3. **Judgemental reflection**—evaluation of the perception, thoughts, behaviours, attitudes

Corresponding Reflective Activity
- Exploration of value judgements arising from the volunteering experience and how these are impacted by considered evidence/reading/rational discourse?

4. **Conceptual reflection**—self-reflection that can raise doubts about the fact if good, bad, or appropriate concepts were used in understanding and the evaluation process

Corresponding Reflective Activity
- Exploration of new/different understandings of self in light of considered evidence and rational discourse?

5. **Psychic reflection**—acknowledges that humans tend to judge and base their judgement on a limited amount of information

Corresponding Reflective Activity
- Has sufficient evidence/rational discourse allowed for a shift in perspective? Is there a need for supplementary evidence/discourse?

6. **Theoretical reflection**—understanding that the ability to perceive and evaluate thoughts, behaviours, attitudes lies in cultural or psychological assumptions that are taken for granted, and that explains why a personal experience is more acceptable than another perspective that uses more functional criteria of seeing, thinking, or behaviour

Corresponding Reflective Activity
- How has *personal* interaction between volunteer, recipient and others contributed to a shift in meaning perspective than would otherwise occur using unitary sources of evidence and discourse?

teachers work together to explore appropriate volunteering activities at each stage of the curriculum, followed by a period of structured reflection using, for example, narrative, dialogic and critical reflective learning and teaching methods for exploration of the student's experience.

A Co-created Curriculum Model for Nursing

The curriculum model described here combines elements of a spiral approach, within a co-created framework. The model emphasises activities and effects, as opposed to plans and intentions, and in this sense, is a process rather than a product model (Neary, 2003). Product models of curriculum design have been criticised for over emphasis on learning objectives and viewed as employing technical, means-to-end reasoning (O'Neill, 2010). While product models can be valuable in developing and communicating transparent outcomes to the student population, the concern with their use in nurse education is for an overemphasis on NMC standards for preregistration nursing, as a prescriptive framework for writing learning outcomes, rather than engaging with students in activities to promote critical thinking skills.

A process model, in contrast, accepts student motivation is an essential element in learning, allowing teachers to reclaim learning outcomes and to frame them more broadly and flexibly (Hussey & Smith, 2003). Process models acknowledge post positivist pedagogy; value the importance of experiential and personal learning, take a socially critical approach to learning and teaching, and use a learner-centred design. Co-creation of the nursing curriculum does not impinge on the need to ensure the curriculum takes account of and meets the requirements set out in the NMC standards for pre-registration nursing. Rather, it pays attention to professional requirements while at the same time acknowledging 'learner as asset', as 'agent for transformational change' and as 'active participants in the learning process'. Figure 7.1 highlights the key differences between product and process curriculum models.

A spiral approach to learning and teaching, predicated on Bruner's cognitive theory, guides the inclusion of content throughout the duration of the nursing programme. Cognitive theory is predicated on the idea

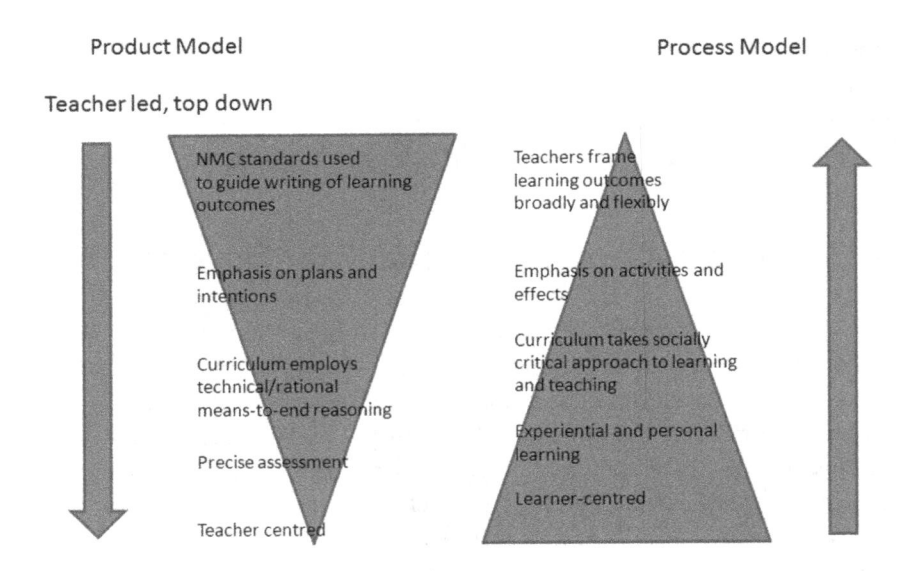

7 Preparing Nurses for Contemporary Nursing Practice

Product Model

Teacher led, top down

- NMC standards used to guide writing of learning outcomes
- Emphasis on plans and intentions
- Curriculum employs technical/rational means-to-end reasoning
- Precise assessment
- Teacher centred

Process Model

- Teachers frame learning outcomes broadly and flexibly
- Emphasis on activities and effects
- Curriculum takes socially critical approach to learning and teaching
- Experiential and personal learning
- Learner-centred

Student centred, bottom up

Fig. 7.1 Product/Process Curriculum Models

that complex material can be more readily understood if structured properly. By using a spiral model specific nursing content can be revisited throughout the curriculum, whereby the levels of complexity increase with each visit. A spiral curriculum design such as this facilitates reinforcement, solidification and logical progression of knowledge. Students are introduced to concepts in nursing at increasing levels of complexity throughout the curriculum, with corresponding increases in complexity in application of theory to practice. Bruner (1960) argued each element of new learning about a topic bears a relationship to previous learning, and is contextualised within previous learning. While clear empirical evidence to link the spiral curriculum to improved student learning is limited, a spiral curriculum recognises the importance of contextualisation of learning in nursing, while at the same time facilitating mastery of fundamental and higher-order nursing competencies. Figure 7.2 illustrates how a spiral design can be used to organise curriculum content across a 3-year undergraduate nursing programme.

Spiral Curriculum Model
(Bruner, 1960)

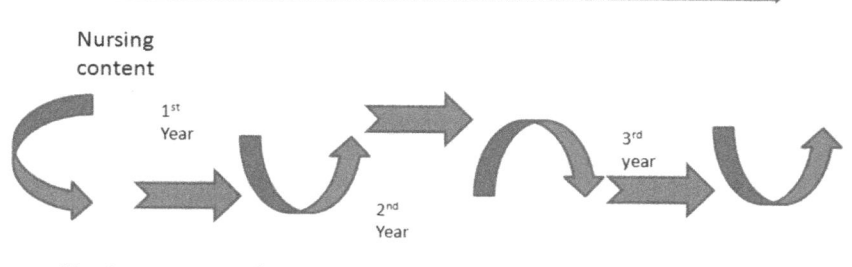

Nursing content

1st Year

2nd Year

3rd year

Nursing content and concepts introduced and revisited in increasing levels of complexity

Fig. 7.2 Spiral Curriculum Model

In addition to a theory of cognition, the co-created model draws on a theory of constructivism, in that student nurses are guided to construct new ideas or concepts in nursing based on current and past knowledge—one example, although not exclusive, being teachers using narrative, dialogic and critical reflective pedagogy to explore volunteering experiences with students. Using constructivist theory to frame the curriculum allows the learner to select and transform information, construct hypotheses, and to make decisions about care, within a safe environment. Within a cognitive structure, the curriculum, underpinned by constructivism becomes meaningful to learners and teachers and allows individual students to go beyond the information provided, to make sense of the realities of nursing practice. Figure 7.3 describes how a process curriculum model, when used in combination with a spiral design allows for the inclusion of broad as opposed to narrowly defined learning outcomes, which subsequently determine learning and teaching in theory and in practice settings. A combined model such as this enables a socially critical approach to learning and teaching, which prioritises a learner-centred approach and legitimises experiential and personal learning.

The combined model described here facilitates the use of a range of transformative pedagogies, for example critical, narrative, dialogic and

Spiral Curriculum Model (Bruner, 1960)

Nursing content and concepts introduced and revisited in increasing levels of complexity

1st Year
2nd Year
3rd year

Process Model (Hussey and Smith, 2003)
Broad learning outcomes. Socially critical approach to learning and teaching. Experiential and personal learning. Learner-centred.

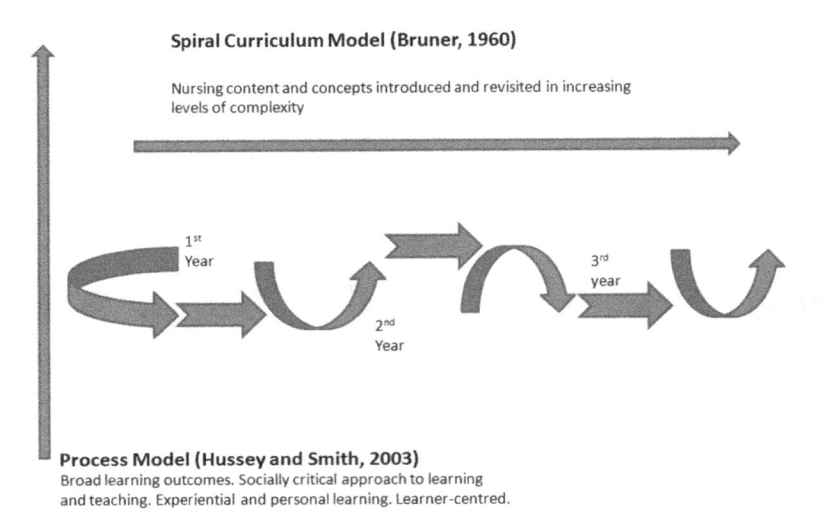

Fig. 7.3 Combined Process/Spiral Curriculum Model

constructivist. Choice of pedagogical approach to learning and teaching is determined by curriculum content, which in turn takes account of individual learner needs. The combined model recognises learners bring their personal histories and life experiences to the curriculum, and that these will change over time as the nursing programme progresses. Figure 7.4 illustrates how the inclusion of volunteering opportunities, followed by structured reflection using narrative, dialogic and critical reflective pedagogies, assists students to construct new knowledge about nursing. Extending the model beyond initial education facilitates the process of life-long learning, while delivering the model alongside professions associated with nursing (medicine, midwifery, physiotherapy, occupational therapy, operating department assistant) facilitates interprofessional and/or multidisciplinary learning and teaching.

Whatever theoretical position is taken towards curriculum development in nursing, and whichever approach is taken to design and subsequently delivery of the nursing curriculum, success will depend on whether or not the gap between rhetoric and reality is addressed. In other words, the theory/practice gap in curriculum development deserves as much attention as the more often quoted theory/practice gap in nurse

A process model for the nursing curriculum
Broad learning outcomes. Socially critical approach to learning and teaching. Experiential and personal learning. Learner-centred.

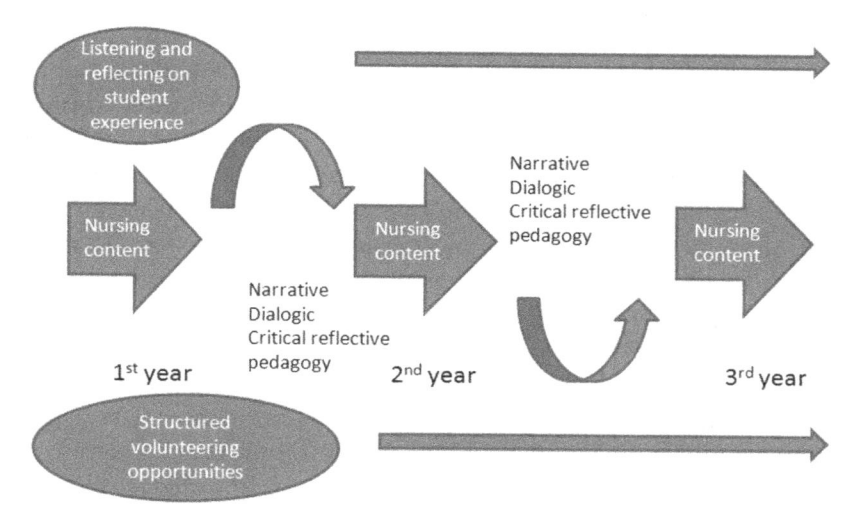

A spiral design to the organisation of nursing content
Nursing content and concepts introduced and revisited in increasing levels of complexity

Fig. 7.4 Volunteering as Pedagogy in a Combined Process/Spiral Curriculum Model

education. A lack of resources in terms of time, and availability of academic staff with the necessary expertise and knowledge often drives curriculum development and determines the outcome, in terms of what the curriculum looks like, its vision, intentions and purposes. With this in mind, experienced nurse academics charged with leading curriculum development need to identify any shortfalls in theoretical and practical knowledge of curriculum development, and take the necessary steps to address any apparent theory/practice gap. As is often the case in curriculum development in nursing, skills are prioritised over knowledge for very good reasons. The need to ensure nursing students achieve a given set of competencies requires teachers with the skills to *teach to competency*, and as such is a powerful driver in curriculum design. Nevertheless, as Paulo Freire points out, "praxis requires theory to illuminate it" (Freire, 1972, p. 96).

The Future for Nurse Education

To suggest nursing is synonymous with change is to understate the case. What nurses do, and how and where they do it is impacted by multiple factors, all of which have been discussed in this book. Changing population demographics, changing patterns of disease and ill health, advancing technology, access to information, rising public expectation, political and economic uncertainty, and shifting ideological beliefs about healthcare all affect the scope of nursing and midwifery practice. It necessarily follows that nurse education has to change to ensure nurses and midwives can adapt to rapidly changing situations and to take on new and complex roles, as and when the need arises. The nursing curriculum needs also to be responsive to change, which requires nurse educators to have the necessary knowledge and skills to shape a dynamic and responsive curriculum, as opposed to a reactive curriculum. However, as previously stated nursing lecturers are often drawn from practice for reasons that clinical expertise is prioritised over and above knowledge of theories and practice in education; more specifically in curriculum development. The resulting curriculum, irrespective of engagement of practitioners in curriculum development embodies education as *product*, with the result that *educating for competency* becomes the dominant learning and teaching strategy. While this approach fulfils the regulatory requirements contained within the standards for pre-registration nursing education, nevertheless the curriculum effectively perpetuates the theory/practice gap in nursing. In the absence of a nursing curriculum conceptualised as praxis the hidden issues, such as working conditions, politics of nursing, inequalities and injustices in health and social care can remain hidden from students, and in this sense, the nursing curriculum does nurse education a disservice, while also going some way towards explaining the high level of attrition of newly qualified nurses from the profession.

One way forward for nurse education is to understand the nursing curriculum in context, whereby what nurses think is given as much priority as what nurses do (Ironside, 2004). The nursing curriculum, considered within the context of the wider issues facing nursing requires a broader consideration of learning and teaching strategies than is possible when the curriculum is conceptualised as product. While the key role of nurse education clearly is to prepare competent practitioners, it must also acknowledge its role in providing nurses with the skills to challenge assumptions, and to articulate when and why care is falling short of standards in order that mitigating contextual factors impacting nursing work are recognised. Narrative, dialogic, critical reflective practice, and consideration of alternative experiences such as those provided by volunteering are examples of pedagogies, which have potential to transform learning and teaching about nursing.

While this book has concentrated on undergraduate nurse education, with little discussion of postgraduate study and/or career pathways for qualified nurses, it is recognised that these are intrinsically linked, with learning about nursing clearly a life-long process. Similarly, interprofessional learning has not been considered, but is recognised as an important consideration in nurse education. Interprofessional learning can be used interchangeably with interdisciplinary education, shared learning, multiprofessional learning (MPL) and transprofessional education. However, all manifestations of interprofessional learning lay claim to a philosophy of collaboration, team working and learning together (Suwaileh & Gwele, 2005). It therefore makes sense for interprofessional learning to feature strongly in nurse education, and in ongoing development of the nursing curriculum. The fact that interprofessional learning can be incorporated across pre- and post-registration programmes makes it ideally placed to impact life-long learning in nursing. A number of considerations are worthy of note, however, when considering approaches to interprofessional learning in the undergraduate nursing curriculum, for example the relationships among various professional groups, professional identities, prejudices, stereotypical views of each other's professions, and the historical status and knowledge base of each of the professions involved. Notwithstanding these considerations, interprofessional learning has potential to enhance teaching and learning about nursing, for reasons that the ultimate goal is to enhance the practice of all the disciplines involved to the mutual benefit of the professions.

Conclusion

The future for undergraduate nurse education, in terms of whether or not nursing remains as a discipline taught within higher education or whether other modes of education or training prevail, depends to a large extent on how nursing is conceptualised. In this book nursing has been conceptualised as art, as science and as a personal and moral commitment. While no single pedagogical approach can be considered instrumental in achieving the recommendations laid out by Sir Robert Francis, nevertheless carefully designed and facilitated nursing curricula enables students to develop critical thinking skills; achieve clinical nursing competencies, while also fostering the behaviours synonymous with caring and compassionate practice.

Conceptualisation of nursing as art, as science and as a personal and moral commitment requires a model for nurse education, which draws on appropriate forms of nursing knowledge and allows for alternative and transformative pedagogies to guide approaches to learning and teaching. While these ideas are not new, nevertheless a process model enables co-creation to underpin approaches to learning and teaching, with learners being recognised as an essential element in determining learning outcomes. A spiral curriculum framework underpinned by cognitive and constructivist theory ensures students achieve both the competencies and intrinsic values underpinning nursing practice.

Co-creation in nurse education is premised on principles of students as assets for learning and teaching, as participants in their learning and teaching journeys, and as agents for transformation and change. In this sense, student nurses are the beneficiaries of nurse education; and as such have capacity, are special, and can contribute to the nursing curriculum in ways they are very rarely asked to do. Nurse educators are similarly integral to the co-creative process, for reasons that as both nurse and teacher they are ideally placed to work together in equal partnership with clinical practitioners to share information, aspirations, and ideas as to what the nursing curriculum should look like. It is in this manner that the nursing curriculum is conceptualised as *praxis* and comes to embody *praxis*. Working within the framework of the Nursing and Midwifery

Council's regulatory requirements should not prevent all those involved in planning, designing and delivering undergraduate nursing programmes from drawing on appropriate transformative pedagogies and considering the co-creation imperative in nurse education.

References

Ailey, S., Lamb, K., Friese, T., & Christopher, B. (2015). Educating nursing students in clinical leadership. *Nursing Management, 21*(9), 23–28.

Bell, K., Tanner, J., Rutty, J., Astley-Pepper, M., & Hall, R. (2014). Successful partnerships with third sector organisations to enhance the student experience: A partnership evaluation. *Nurse Education Today, 33*(3), 530–534.

Benner, P., Tanner, C., & Chesla, C. (2009). *Expertise in nursing practice* (2nd ed.). New York: Springer.

Benton, D. (2011). Nurses fit for purpose, award and practice? *International Nursing Review, 58*(3), 276.

Blanchet Garneau, A., Browne, A. J., & Varcoe, C. (2016). *Integrating social justice in health care curriculum: Drawing on antiracist approaches toward a critical antidiscriminatory pedagogy for nursing* (2nd ed.). Sydney: International Critical Perspectives in Nursing and Healthcare.

Britnell, M. (2015). *In search of the perfect health system*. London: Palgrave Macmillan.

Bruner, J. S. (1960). *The process of education*. Cambridge, MA: Harvard University Press.

Council for Healthcare and Regulatory Excellence. (2012). *Strategic review of the nursing and midwifery council: Final report*. London: CHRE.

Dyson, S. E., Liu, L. Q., van den Akker, O., & O'Driscoll, M. (2017). The extent, variability and attitudes towards volunteering among undergraduate nursing students: Implications for pedagogy in nurse education. *Nurse Education in Practice, 23*, 15–22.

Freire, P. (1972). *Pedagogy of the oppressed*. London: Penguin Books.

Furnham, A. (2014). Why go to university? Retrieved May 17, 2017, from https://www.psychologytoday.com/blog/sideways-view/201403/why-go-university

Grundy, S. (1987). *Curriculum: Product or praxis?* Lewes: Falmer Press.

Hafford-Letchfield, T., Thomas, B., & McDonald, L. (2016). Social work students as community partners in a family intervention programme. *Journal of Social Work*, 1–20. ISSN 1468-0173. Published online first.

Ham, C., Dixon, A., & Brooke, B. (2012). *Transforming the delivery of health and social care: The case for fundamental change*. London: The King's Fund.

Hussey, T., & Smith, P. (2003). The uses of learning outcomes. *Teaching in Higher Education, 8*(3), 357–368.

Ironside, P. M. (2004). "Covering content" and teaching thinking: Deconstructing the additive curriculum. *Journal of Nursing Education, 43*(1), 5–12.

Ironside, P. M. (2006). Using narrative pedagogy: Learning and practising interpretive thinking. *Journal of Advanced Nursing, 55*(4), 478–486.

John, P. D. (2006). Lesson planning and the student teacher: Re-thinking the dominant model. *Journal of Curriculum Studies, 38*(4), 483–498.

Jones, S., & Hill, K. (2003). Understanding patterns of commitment: Motivation for community service involvement. *Journal of Higher Education, 74*(5), 516–539.

Kelly, A. V. (2009). *The curriculum: Theory and practice* (6th ed.). London: Sage.

Lave, J., & Wenger, E. (1991). *Situated learning: Legitimate peripheral participation*. Cambridge: Cambridge University Press.

McAllister, M. (2010). Awake and aware: Thinking constructively about the world through transformative learning. In T. Warne & S. McAndrew (Eds.), *Creative approaches to health and social care education: Knowing me, understanding you*. Basingstoke: Palgrave Macmillan.

McBride, A., & Lough, B. (2010). Access to international volunteering. *Nonprofit Management and Leadership, 21*(2), 195–208.

McSherry, W. (2013). Do nurses care? Retrieved May 18, 2017, from https://blog.oup.com/2013/05/do-nurses-care/

Mezirow, J. (1991). *Transformative dimensions of adult learning*. San Francisco: Jossey Bass.

Morrow-Howell, N. (2010). Volunteering in later life: Research frontiers. *Journals of Gerontology Series B Psychological Sciences and Social Sciences, 65*(4), 461–469.

Mundle, C., Naylor, C., & Buck, D. (2012). Volunteering in health and care in England: A summary of key literature. *The King's Fund*, London. Retrieved July 19, 2016, from www.kingsfund.org.uk/sites/files/kt/field/field_realted_document/volunteering-in-health-literature-review-kingsfund-mar13.pdf

Neary, M. (2003). Curriculum models and developments in adult education. In *Curriculum studies in post-compulsory and adult education: A teacher's and student teacher's study guide*. Cheltenham: Nelson Thornes Ltd.

O'Neill, G. (2010). Initiating curriculum revision: Exploring the practices of educational developers. *International Journal for Academic Development, 15*(1), 61–71.

Paylor, J. (2011). *Volunteering and health: Evidence of impact and implications for policy and practice.* London: Institute for Volunteering Research.

Ravi, V. (2016). *Curriculum development.* Raleigh: Lulu Publications.

RCN. (2014, March 31). *Response of the Royal College of Nursing to the Nursing and Midwifery Council consultation on revalidation.* London: RCN.

Renigere, R. (2014). Transformative learning in the discipline of nursing. *American Journal of Educational Research, 2*(12), 1207–1210.

Reyes, H., Hadley, L., & Davenport, D. (2013). A comparative analysis of cultural competence in beginning and graduating nursing students. *ISRN Nursing,* 929764. doi:10.1155/2013/929764

Rumay Alexander, G. (2008). Cultural competence models in nursing. *Critical Care Nursing Clinics of North America, 20,* 415–421.

Scott, H. (2004). Are nurses too clever to care' and too posh to wash. *British Journal of Nursing, 13*(10), 581.

Sheehan, J. (1986). Curriculum models: Product versus process. *Journal of Advanced Nursing, 11,* 671–678.

Smith, M. K. (2000). Curriculum theory and practice. *The Encyclopaedia of Informal Education.* Retrieved May 22, 2017, from http://infed.org/mobi/curriculum-theory-and=practice/

Stenhouse, L. (1975). *An introduction to curriculum research and development.* London: Heinemann.

Suwaileh, M., & Gwele, N. S. (2005). A curriculum for interprofessional learning. In L. R. Uys & N. S. Gwele (Eds.), *Curriculum development in nursing: Process and innovations.* London: Routledge.

References

About Dialogue Education. (n.d.). Retrieved July 19, 2016, from http://www.globallearningpartners.com/about/about-dialogue-education

Aiken, L. H., Buchan, J., Sochalski, J., Nichols, B., & Powell, M. (2004). Trends in international nurse migration. *Health Affairs, 23*(3), 69–77.

Ailey, S., Lamb, K., Friese, T., & Christopher, B. (2015). Educating nursing *students* in clinical leadership. *Nursing Management, 21*(9), 23–28.

Aldrich, R. (2006). *Lessons from history of education*. London: Routledge.

Alexander, R. (2000). Towards dialogic teaching. Retrieved May 27, 2017, from www.robinalexander.org.uk

Allan, H. T., & Larsen, J. A. (2003). *"We need respect": Experiences of internationally recruited nurses in the UK*. London: RCN.

Appleby, J. (2016). How does NHS spending compare with health spending internationally? Retrieved April 24, 2017, from https://www.kingsfund.org.uk/blog/2016/01/how-does-nhs-spending-compare-health-spending-internationally

Baker, E. (2015). Transparency will only change culture if we eradicate blame as a response. Retrieved December 9, 2016, from http://www.cqc.org.uk/content/transparency-will-only-change-culture-if-we-eradicate-blame-response

Ball, J. E., Murrells, T., Rafferty, A., Morrow, E., & Griffiths, P. (2013, July 29). Care left undone during nursing shifts: Associations with workload and perceived quality of care. *BMJ Quality and Safety*, Online First. Retrieved November 30, 2016, from http://qualitysafety.bmj.com/

Bell, K., Tanner, J., Rutty, J., Astley-Pepper, M., & Hall, R. (2014). Successful partnerships with third sector organisations to enhance the student experience: A partnership evaluation. *Nurse Education Today, 33*(3), 530–534.

Benner, P., Tanner, C., & Chesla, C. (2009). *Expertise in nursing practice* (2nd ed.). New York: Springer.

Benton, D. (2011). Nurses fit for purpose, award and practice? *International Nursing Review, 58*(3), 276.

Bernstein, B. (1971). *Class, codes and control* (Vol. 1). London: Kegan Paul.

Betancourt, L. A., Ostrom, A. L., Brown, S. W., & Roundtree, R. I. (2002). Client co-production in knowledge-intensive business services. *California Management Review, 44*, 100–128.

Bewley, A. (2016). Is education to blame for safeguarding failures. *Nursing Standard, 30*(19), 32–33.

Blanchet Garneau, A. (2016). Critical reflection in cultural competence development: A framework for undergraduate nursing education. *Journal of Nursing Education, 55*(3), 125–132.

Blanchet Garneau, A., Browne, A. J., & Varcoe, C. (2016). *Integrating social justice in health care curriculum: Drawing on antiracist approaches toward a critical antidiscriminatory pedagogy for nursing* (2nd ed.). Sydney: International Critical Perspectives in Nursing and Healthcare.

Bloom, B., Englehart, M., Furst, E., Hill, W., & Krathwohl, D. (1956). *Taxonomy of educational objectives: The classification of educational goals. Handbook I: Cognitive domain.* New York, Toronto: Longmans, Green.

Boeck, T., Makadia, N., Johnson, C., Cadogan, N., Salim, H., & Cushing, J. (2009). The impact of volunteering on social capital and community cohesion. Retrieved July 18, 2016, from http://www.dmu.ac.uk/documents/health-and-life-sciences-documents/centre-for-social-action/research/project-reaction-final-report.pdf

Boud, D., Keogh, R., & Walker, D. (1985). *Reflection: Turning experience into learning.* London: Kogan Page.

Bourdieu, P., & Wacquant, L. J. D. (1992). *An invitation to reflexive sociology.* Chicago: University of Chicago Press.

Bovill, C. (2013). Students and staff co-creating curricula: A new trend or an old idea we never got around to implementing? In C. Rust (Ed.), *Improving student learning through research and scholarship: 20 years of ISL, Improving student learning (20). Oxford Centre for Staff and Learning Development* (pp. 96–108). Oxford: OCSD.

Bovill, C., Cook-Sather, A., & Felten, P. (2011). Changing participants in pedagogical planning: Students as co-creators of teaching approaches, course design and curricula. *International Journal of Academic Development, 16*(2), 133–145.

Boyle, D., & Harris, M. (2009). *The challenge of co-production: How equal partnerships between professionals and the public are crucial to improving public services*. Discussion paper, NESTA, London.

BPP. (2016). The apprenticeship levy – Opportunities for your business. Retrieved December 2, 2016, from www.bpp.com

Bratanova, B., Loughnan, S., Klein, O., & Wood, R. (2016). The rich get richer, the poor get even: Perceived socio-economic position influences micro-social distribution of wealth. *Scandinavian Journal of Psychology, 57*(3), 243–249.

Britnell, M. (2015). *In search of the perfect health system*. London: Palgrave Macmillan.

Bruner, J. S. (1960). *The process of education*. Cambridge, MA: Harvard University Press.

Bryk, A. S., & Schneider, B. (2002). *Trust in schools: A core resource for improvement*. New York, NY: Russell Sage Foundation.

Cahn, E. S. (2004). *No more throw-away people: The co-production imperative* (1st ed.). Washington, DC: Essential Books.

Campbell, D. (2016). NHS hospitals in England reveal £2.45 bn record deficit. Retrieved from http://www.theguardian.com/society/2016/may/20/nhs-in-england-reveals-245bn-record-deficit

Carper, B. A. (1978). Fundamental patterns of knowing in nursing. *Advances in Nursing Science, 1*(1), 13–24.

Carr, S. (2014). *Guide to co-production in mental health and social care*. Community Care Inform Adults (online resource).

Chattoo, S., & Ahmad, W. I. U. (2008). The moral economy of selfhood and caring: Negotiating boundaries of personal care as embodied moral practice. *Sociology of Health & Illness, 30*(4), 550–564.

Chelf, J. H., Deshler, A. M. B., Hillman, S., & Durazo-Arvizu, R. (2000). Storytelling: A strategy for coping with cancer. *Cancer Nursing, 23*(1), 1–5.

Cipriano, P. (2007). Celebrating the art and science of nursing. *American Nurse Today, 2*(5), 8.

Coles, T. (2014). Critical pedagogy: Schools must equip students to challenge the status quo. Retrieved December 13, 2016, from https://www.theguardian.com/teacher-network/teacher-blog/2014/feb/25/critical-pedagogy-schools-students-challenge

References

Cooper, Z., Gibbon, S., Jones, S., & McGuire, A. (2011). Does hospital competition save lives? Evidence from the English NHS patient choice reforms. *The Economic Journal, 121*(554), F228–F260.

Corrie, C., & Mosseri-Marlio, W. (2015). *Progress on NHS reform*. London: Reform.

Council for Healthcare and Regulatory Excellence. (2012). *Strategic review of the nursing and midwifery council: Final report*. London: CHRE.

Council of Deans of Health. (2016). Educating the future nurse – A paper for discussion. Retrieved November 9, 2016, from www.councilofdeans.org.uk

CQC. (2016). Retrieved from http://www.cqc.org.uk/content/special-measures

Denscombe, M. (2008). Communities of practice: A research paradigm for the mixed methods approach. *Journal of Mixed Methods Research, 2*(3), 270–283.

Dewey, J. (1900). The psychology of the elementary curriculum. Cited by Plagens, G. (2011). Social capital and education: Implications for student and school performance. *E&C/Education &Culture, 27*(1): 40–64.

Dewey, J. (1938). Experience and education. Retrieved December 13, 2016, from http://ruby.fgcu.edu/courses/ndemers/colloquium/experienceeducationdewey.pdf

Diekelmann, N. (2001). Narrative pedagogy: Heideggerian hermeneutical analyses of lived experiences of students, teachers, and clinicians. *Advances in Nursing Science, 23*(3), 53–71.

Dyson, S. E., Liu, L. Q., van den Akker, O., & O'Driscoll, M. (2017). The extent, variability and attitudes towards volunteering among undergraduate nursing students: Implications for pedagogy in nurse education. *Nurse Education in Practice, 23*, 15–22.

Eaton, A. (2012). Pre-registration nurse education: A brief history. Retrieved December 8, 2016, from www.willliscommission.org.uk

Edwards, S. (2002). Nursing knowledge: Defining new boundaries (art and science development). *Nursing Standard, 17*(2), 40–44.

Ennis, R. H. (1987). Critical thinking and the curriculum. In M. Heiman & J. Slominanko (Eds.), *Thinking skills instruction: Concepts and techniques*. Washington, DC: National Education Association.

Escotet, M. A. (2012). *There is today a need to educate for uncertainty*. The Escotet Foundation. Retrieved June 5, 2016, from http://escotet.org/2014/01/today-there-is-a-need-to-educate-for-uncertainty/

Fielding, M. (1999). Radical collegiality: Affirming teaching as an inclusive professional practice. *Australian Educational Researcher, 26*(2), 1–34.

Francis, R. (2013). *Report of the Mid Staffordshire NHS Foundation Trust public inquiry*. London: The Stationery Office.

Fraser, S., & Bosanquet, A. (2006). The curriculum? That's just a unit outline, isn't it? *Studies in Higher Education, 31*(3), 269–284.

Freire, P. (1972). *Pedagogy of the oppressed*. London: Penguin Books.

Freire, P. (1985). Reading the world and reading the word: An interview with Paulo Freire. *Language Arts, 62*(1), 15–21.

Furnham, A. (2014). Why go to university? Retrieved May 17, 2017, from https://www.psychologytoday.com/blog/sideways-view/201403/why-go-university

Ganly, S. (2016). Educational philosophies in the classroom. Retrieved November 9, 2016, from www.doe.in.gov>cte>ncteb-edphil

Giroux, H. A. (2006). Higher education under siege: Implications for public intellectuals. *The NEA Higher Education Journal*, Fall, 63–78.

Giroux, H. A. (2011). *On critical pedagogy*. New York: Bloomsbury.

Gov.UK. (2014). Guidance: Future of apprenticeships in England: Guidance for trailblazers. Department for Business, Innovation & Skills and Department for Education. Retrieved from https://www.gov.uk/government/publications/future-of-apprenticeships-in-england-guidance-for-trailblazers

Gov.UK. (2016). Transparency data: NHS foundation trust directory. Retrieved from https://www.gov.uk/government/publications/nhs-foundation-trust-directory/nhs-foundation-trust-directory

Grosios, K., Gahan, P. B., & Burbidge, J. (2010). Overview of healthcare in the UK. *The EPMA Journal, 1*(4), 529–534.

Grow, G. O. (1991). Cited in Wang, V. C. X., & Sarbo, L. (2004). Philosophy, role of adult educators, and learning. How contextually adapted philosophies and the situational role of adult educators affect learners' transformation and emancipation. *Journal of Transformative Education, 2*(3): 204–214.

Grundy, S. (1987). *Curriculum: Product or praxis?* Lewes: Falmer Press.

Hafford-Letchfield, T., & Lavender, P. (2015). Quality improvement through the paradigm of learning. *Quality in Ageing and Older Adults, 16*(4), 1–13.

Hafford-Letchfield, T., Thomas, B., & McDonald, L. (2016). Social work students as community partners in a family intervention programme. *Journal of Social Work*, 1–20. ISSN 1468-0173. Published online first.

Hall, C. (2004, May 11). Young nurses "too posh to wash". *The Telegraph*. Retrieved December 21, 2016, from http://www.telegraph.co.uk/news/uknews/1461504/Young-nurses-too-posh-to-wash.html

References

Ham, C., Dixon, A., & Brooke, B. (2012). *Transforming the delivery of health and social care: The case for fundamental change.* London: The King's Fund.

Heaslip, P. (1993). Revised 2008 critical thinking and nursing. Retrieved May 9, 2017, from http://www.criticalthinking.org/pages/critical-thinking-and-nursing/834

HEE. (2016). Values based recruitment framework. Health Education England. Retrieved December 9, 2016, from https://www.hee.nhs.uk/.../values-based-recruitment

Hicks, S. (2004). *Explaining postmodernism: Skepticism and socialism from Rousseau to Foucault* (pp. 18–19). Tempe, AZ: Scholargy Press.

Higher Education Academy. (2017). Learning through storytelling. Retrieved May 28, 2017, from https://www.heacademy.ac.uk/enhancement/starter-tools/learning-through-storytelling

Hughes, A. J., & Fraser, D. M. (2011). "SINK or SWIM": The experience of newly qualified midwives in England. *Midwifery, 27*(3), 382–386.

Hughes, R. G. (2008). Nurses at the "sharp end" of patient care. In R. G. Hughes (Ed.), *Patient safety and quality: An evidence-based handbook for nurses.* Rockville, MD: AHRQ Publishers.

Hunt. (2013). Cited in Department of Health press release. Hunt sets out tough new to turn around NHS hospitals. Retrieved from https://www.gov.uk/government/news/hunt-sets-out-tough-new-approach-to-turn-around-nhs-hospitals

Hussey, T., & Smith, P. (2003). The uses of learning outcomes. *Teaching in Higher Education, 8*(3), 357–368.

Ironside, P. M. (2001). Creating a research base for nursing education: An interpretive review of conventional, critical, feminist, postmodern, and phenomenologic pedagogies. *Advances in Nursing Science, 23*(3), 72–87.

Ironside, P. M. (2003). New pedagogies for teaching thinking: The lived experiences of students and teachers enacting narrative pedagogy. *Journal of Nursing Education, 42,* 509–516.

Ironside, P. M. (2004). "Covering content" and teaching thinking: Deconstructing the additive curriculum. *Journal of Nursing Education, 43*(1), 5–12.

Ironside, P. M. (2006). Using narrative pedagogy: Learning and practising interpretive thinking. *Journal of Advanced Nursing, 55*(4), 478–486.

Ironside, P. M. (2014). Enabling narrative pedagogy: Inviting, waiting and letting-be. *Nursing Education Perspectives, 35*(3), 212–218.

Ironside, P. M. (2015). Narrative pedagogy: Transforming nursing education through of research. *Nursing Education Perspectives, 36*(2), 83–88.

Ironside, P. M., & Hayden-Miles, M. (2012). Narrative pedagogy: Co-creating engaging learning experiences with students. In G. Sherwood & S. Horton-Deutsch (Eds.), *Reflective practice: Transforming education and improving outcomes* (pp. 135–148). Indianapolis, IN: Sigma Theta Tau International.

James, N. (1992). Care = organisation + physical labour + emotional labour. *Sociology of Health & Illness, 14*, 488–509.

John, P. D. (2006). Lesson planning and the student teacher: Re-thinking the dominant model. *Journal of Curriculum Studies, 38*(4), 483–498.

Jones, S., & Hill, K. (2003). Understanding patterns of commitment: Motivation for community service involvement. *Journal of Higher Education, 74*(5), 516–539.

Kamradt-Scott, A. (2015). WHO's to blame? The World Health Organization and the 2014 Ebola outbreak in West Africa. *Third World Quarterly, 32*(3), 401. The international politics of Ebola.

Kapur, N. (2014). Mid Staffordshire Hospital report: What does psychology have to offer. *The Psychologist, 27*, 16–20.

Karimi, Z., Ashktourab, T., Mohammadi, M., & Ali Abedi, H. (2014). Using the hidden curriculum to teach professionalism in nursing students. *Iranian Red Crescent Medical Journal, 16*(3), e15532.

Kelly, A. V. (2009). *The curriculum: Theory and practice* (6th ed.). London: Sage.

Killingley, J., & Dyson, S. E. (2016). Student midwives' perspectives on efficacy of feedback after structured clinical examination. *British Journal of Midwifery, 24*(5), 362–368.

Kuhn, T. (1970). *The structure of scientific revolutions*. Chicago: University of Chicago Press.

Lave, J., & Wenger, E. (1991). *Situated learning: Legitimate peripheral participation*. Cambridge: Cambridge University Press.

Lewis, N. (2003). World health organization profile: Criticisms of WHO. Retrieved April 26, 2017, from http://health.howstuffworks.com/medicine/health/care/who5.htm

Macleod Clark, J. (2016). *Developing new standards for the future graduate registered nurse*. Council of Deans. Retrieved April 25, 2017, from https://councilofdeans.org.uk/2016/08/developing-new-standards-for-the-future-graduate-registered-nurse/

Maguire, D., Dunn, P., & Mckenna, H. (2016). How hospital activity in the NHS in England has changed over time. Retrieved May 3, 2017, from https://www.kingsfund.org.uk/publications/hospital-activity-funding-changes

References

Malsher, A. (2013). Duty of candour: Patients deserve more protection than simple contracts. Retrieved from https://www.theguardian.com/healthcare-network/2013/apr/03/nhs-reforms-duty-of-candour-mid-staffs-scandal

Martin, J. S., Ummenhofer, W., Manser, T., & Spirig, R. (2010). Interprofessional collaboration among nurses and physicians: Making a difference in patient outcomes. *Swiss Medical Weekly, 140*, w13062.

Mason, M. (2008). *Critical thinking and learning*. Oxford: Blackwell Publishing.

Masters, K., & Gibbs, T. (2007). The spiral curriculum: Implications for on-line learning. *BMC Medical Education, 7*(1), 52.

McAllister, M. (2010). Awake and aware: Thinking constructively about the world through transformative learning. In T. Warne & S. McAndrew (Eds.), *Creative approaches to health and social care education: Knowing me, understanding you*. Basingstoke: Palgrave Macmillan.

McBride, A., & Lough, B. (2010). Access to international volunteering. *Nonprofit Management and Leadership, 21*(2), 195–208.

McKenna, H. (2016). Five big issues for health and social care after the Brexit vote. Retrieved April 24, 2017, from https://www.kingsfund.org.uk/publications/articles/brexit-and-nhs

McLaren, P. (2009). Critical pedagogy: A look at the major concepts. In A. Darder, M. P. Baltodarno, & R. D. Torres (Eds.), *The critical pedagogy reader* (2nd ed.). New York: Routledge.

McLean, M. (2008). *Pedagogy and the university: Critical theory and practice*. London: Continuum.

McSherry, W. (2013). Do nurses care? Retrieved May 18, 2017, from https://blog.oup.com/2013/05/do-nurses-care/

Mezirow, J. (1978). Perspective transformation. *Adult Education, 28*(2), 100–110.

Mezirow, J. (1991). *Transformative dimensions of adult learning*. San Francisco: Jossey Bass.

Mezirow, J. (1997). Transformative learning: Theory to practice. *New Directions for Adult and Continuing Education, 74*, 5–12.

Morrow-Howell, N. (2010). Volunteering in later life: Research frontiers. *Journals of Gerontology Series B Psychological Sciences and Social Sciences, 65*(4), 461–469.

Mundle, C., Naylor, C., & Buck, D. (2012). Volunteering in health and care in England: A summary of key literature. *The King's Fund*, London. Retrieved July 19, 2016, from www.kingsfund.org.uk/sites/files/kt/field/field_realted_document/volunteering-in-health-literature-review-kingsfund-mar13.pdf

Myers, M. G., Godwin, M., Kiss, A., Tobe, S., Curry Grant, F., & Kaczorowski, J. (2011). Conventional versus automated measurement of blood pressure in primary care patients with systolic hypertension: Randomised parallel design controlled trial. *BMJ, 342*, d286. doi:10.1136/bmj.d286

Neary, M. (2003). Curriculum models and developments in adult education. In *Curriculum studies in post-compulsory and adult education: A teacher's and student teacher's study guide*. Cheltenham: Nelson Thornes Ltd.

Needham, C. (2009). SCIE Research briefing 31: Co-production: An emerging evidence base for adult social care transformation. Retrieved July 18, 2016, from http://www.scie.org.uk/publications/briefings/briefing31/

Needham, C., & Carr, S. (2002). SCIE Research Briefing 31: Co-production: An emerging evidence base for adult social care transformation. London: Social Care Institute for Excellence. Retrieved from www.scie.org.co

NHS Atlas of Variation in Healthcare. (2015). Retrieved from http://www.rightcare.nhs.uk/atlas/2015_IAb/atlas.html

NHS England. (2014). Five year forward view. Retrieved June 5, 2016, from https://www.england.nhs.uk/wp-content/uploads/2014/10/5yfv-web.pdf

NHS England. (2017). Next steps on the five year forward view. Retrieved April 24, 2017, from https://www.england.nhs.uk/five-year-forward-view/#

NIH National Institute on Aging. (2011). Longer lives and disability. Retrieved from https://auth.nia.nih.gov/research/publication/global-health-and-aging/longer-lives-and-disability

NMC. (2010). *Standards for pre-registration nursing education*. London: NMC.

NMC. (2013). NMC response to the Francis report. The response of the Nursing and Midwifery Council to the Mid Staffordshire NHS Foundation Trust Public Inquiry report. 18 July 2016. Retrieved December 7, 2016, from http://www.nmc.org.uk/globalassets/sitedocuments/francis-report/nmc-response

NMC. (2015a). *Nursing and midwifery council annual fitness to practise report 2014–2015*, Nursing and Midwifery Council, HMSO, London.

NMC. (2015b). *The code: Professional standards of practice and behaviour for nurses and midwives*. NMC, London. Retrieved from www.nmc-uk.org

NMC. (2016a). Our role in education. Retrieved June 5, 2016, from https://www.nmc.org.uk/education/our-role-in-education/

NMC. (2016b). Revalidation. Retrieved December 9, 2016, from http://revalidation.nmc.org.uk/

Nurses, Midwives and Health Visitors Act. (1979). London: The Stationery Office.

O'Kane, C. E. (2012). Newly qualified nurses' experiences in the intensive care unit. *Nursing in Critical Care, 17*(1), 44–51.

O'Neill, G. (2010). Initiating curriculum revision: Exploring the practices of educational developers. *International Journal for Academic Development, 15*(1), 61–71.

Office for National Statistics (ONS). (2016a). Office for National Statistics (ONS), [GB]. Retrieved from https://www.ons.gov.uk/peoplepopulationandcommunity/birthsdeathsandmarriages/lifeexpectancies/bulletins/pastandprojecteddatafromtheperiodandcohortlifetables/2014baseduk1981to2064#life-expectancy-ex-at-birth-in-the-uk

Office for National Statistics (ONS). (2016b). What works wellbeing. Retrieved July 18, 2016, from https://whatworkswellbeing.org/2016/05/26/social-capital-across-the-uk/

Orton, S. (2011). Re-thinking attrition in student nurses. *Journal of Health and Social Care Improvement., 2011*, 1–7.

Ostrom, E. (1996). Crossing the great divide: Coproduction, synergy, and development. *World Development, 24*(6), 1073–1087.

Pagnucci, N., Carnevale, F., Bagnasco, A., & Sasso, L. F. (2015). A Cross-sectional study of pedagogical strategies in nursing education: Opportunities and constraints toward using effective pedagogy. *BMC Medical Education, 15*, 138.

Paul, R. (1990). *Critical thinking: What every person needs to survive in a rapidly changing world*. Rohnert Park, CA: Center for Critical Thinking and Moral Critique.

Paylor, J. (2011). *Volunteering and health: Evidence of impact and implications for policy and practice*. London: Institute for Volunteering Research.

Peate, I. (2013). *The student nurse toolkit: An essential guide to surviving your course*. Chichester: John Wiley and Sons Ltd.

Pittman, P. (2013). Nursing workforce education, migration and the quality of health care: A global challenge. *International Journal for Quality in Health Care, 25*(4), 349–351.

Price, A. (2004). Encouraging reflection and critical thinking in practice. *Nursing Standard, 18*(47), 46–52.

Proctor, S., Wallbank, S., & Dhaliwal, J. S. (2013). What compassionate care means. Retrieved December 3, 2016, from www.hsj.co.uk/comment/what-compassionate-care-means/5055438.artile

PSA. (2014/2015). *Professional standards for authority for health and social care*. Annual Reports and Accounts and Performance Review Report 2014/2015, PSA, London.

Quality Assurance Agency (QAA). (2015). *The quality code.* Retrieved from www.qaa.ac.uk

Ravi, V. (2016). *Curriculum development.* Raleigh: Lulu Publications.

Ray, M. A. (1991). Caring inquiry: The esthetic process in the way of compassion. In M. C. Smith, M. C. Turkel, & Z. R. Wolf (Eds.), *Caring in nursing classics: An essential resource.* New York: Springer Publishing Company.

RCN. (2003, republished 2014). *Defining nursing.* London: RCN. Online. Retrieved December 3, 2016, from www.rcn.org.uk

RCN. (2013a). *Mid Staffordshire NHS foundation trust: Response of the Royal College of Nursing.* London: RCN. Retrieved from www.rcn.org.uk

RCN. (2013b). *Royal College of Nursing employment survey.* London: RCN. Retrieved from https://www2.rcn.org.uk/__data/assets/pdf_file/0005/541292/Employment_Survey_2013_004_503_FINAL_100214.pdf

RCN. (2014, March 31). *Response of the Royal College of Nursing to the Nursing and Midwifery Council consultation on revalidation.* London: RCN.

RCN. (2016). *What the RCN does.* London: RCN. Retrieved December 7, 2016, from http://www.rcn.org.uk/about-us/what-the-rcn-does

Renigere, R. (2014). Transformative learning in the discipline of nursing. *American Journal of Educational Research, 2*(12), 1207–1210.

Report of the Committee on Nursing. (1972). Chairman: Professor Asa Briggs, Cmnd. 5115, HMSO, London.

Reyes, H., Hadley, L., & Davenport, D. (2013). A comparative analysis of cultural competence in beginning and graduating nursing students. *ISRN Nursing,* 929764. doi:10.1155/2013/929764

Rogers, B. L. (1989). Concepts, analysis and the development of nursing knowledge: The evolutionary cycle. *Journal of Advanced Nursing, 14,* 330–335.

Rumay Alexander, G. (2008). Cultural competence models in nursing. *Critical Care Nursing Clinics of North America, 20,* 415–421.

Salama, A. M. (2009). *Transformative pedagogy in architecture and urbanism.* Solingen: Umbau-Verlag.

Sanders, B. N., & Stappers, P. J. (2008). Co-creation and the new landscapes of design. *CoDesign, 4*(1), 5–18.

Schmitt, T., Sims-Giddens, S., & Booth, R. (2012). Social media use in nursing education. *The Online Journal of Issues in Nursing, 17*(3), 2.

Scott, H. (2004). Are nurses too clever to care' and too posh to wash. *British Journal of Nursing, 13*(10), 581.

Shah, A. (2011). Health care around the world. Retrieved from http://www.globalissues.org/article/774/health-care-around-the-world#TheUSandHealthCare

Shaw, H. K., & Degazon, C. (2008). Integrating the core professional values of nursing: A profession, not just a career. *Journal of Cultural Diversity, 15*(1), 44–50.

Sheehan, J. (1986). Curriculum models: Product versus process. *Journal of Advanced Nursing, 11*, 671–678.

Skeggs, B. (2014). Values beyond value? Is anything beyond the logic of capital? *British Journal of Sociology, 65*(1), 1–20.

Smith, M. K. (2000). Curriculum theory and practice. *The Encyclopaedia of Informal Education*. Retrieved May 22, 2017, from http://infed.org/mobi/curriculum-theory-and=practice/

Smith, M. K. (2002). Jerome Bruner and the process of education. *The Encyclopaedia of Informal Education*. Retrieved July 18, 2016, from http://infed.org/mobi/jerome-bruner-and-the-process-of-education/

Stenhouse, L. (1975). *An introduction to curriculum research and development*. London: Heinemann.

Stiegler, B. (2015). *States of shock: Stupidity and knowledge in the 21st century: Pharmacology of the university*. Cambridge: Polity Press.

Suwaileh, M., & Gwele, N. S. (2005). A curriculum for interprofessional learning. In L. R. Uys & N. S. Gwele (Eds.), *Curriculum development in nursing: Process and innovations*. London: Routledge.

The Cavendish Review. (2013). *An independent review into healthcare assistants and support workers in the NHS and social care settings*. London: Department of Health.

The King's Fund. (2017). Sustainability and transformation plans explained. Retrieved April 25, 2017, from https://www.kingsfund.org.uk/topics/integrated-care/sustainability-transformation-plans-explained

The Nuffield Trust. (2014). The Francis report: One year on. Retrieved December 7, 2016, from www.nuffiledtrust.org.uk

Ukpokodu, O. N. (2009). Pedagogies that foster transformative learning in a multicultural education course: A refection. *Journal of Praxis in Multicultural Education, 4*(1). doi:10.9741/2161-2978.1003

Vallance, E. (1983). Hiding the hidden curriculum: An interpretation of the language of justification in nineteenth-century educational reform. In H. Giroux & D. Purpel (Eds.), *The hidden curriculum and moral education* (pp. 9–27). Berkeley, CA: McCutchan Publishing Corporation.

Vize, R. (2016). Sustainability and transformation plans are 'least bad option' for NHS. Retrieved April 25, 2017, from https://www.theguardian.com/

healthcare-network/2016/oct/21/sustainability-and-transformation-plans-least-bad-option-nhs

Walker, S. (2013). *Mid Staffs: Was it what we've been told?* Retrieved from https://skwalker1964.wordpress.com/2013/02/26/the-real-mid-staffs-story-one-excess-death-if-that/

Wallin, R., Ewald, U., Wikblad, K., Scott-Finley, S., & Arnetz, B. (2006). Understandings work contextual factors: A short-cut to evidence-based practice? *Evidence-Based Nursing, 3*(4), 153–164.

Wang, V. C. X., & Sarbo, L. (2004). Philosophy, role of adult educators, and learning: How contextually adapted philosophies and the situational role of adult educators affects learners' transformation and emancipation. *Journal of Transformative Education, 2*(3), 204–214.

WHO. (2006). *Working together for health*. The World Health Report. The World Health Organisation, Geneva.

WHO. (2009). *Global standards for the initial education of professional nurses and midwives*. Geneva: World Health Organisation.

WHO. (2014). *World health statistics 2014*. Geneva: World Health Organisation.

WHO. (2016a). Global health observatory data. World health statistics 2016: Monitoring health for the SDGs. Retrieved December 14, 2016, from www.who.int/gho/publications/world_health_statistics/2016/en/

WHO. (2016b). *Nurse educator core competencies*. Geneva: World Health Organisation.

WHO. (2017). About WHO: Who we are, what we do. Retrieved from http://www.who.int/about/en/

Willis Commission. (2012). *Quality with compassion: The future of nursing education*. Report of the Willis Commission, London: RCN. Retrieved from www.williscommission.org.uk

Wittek, L., & Kvernbekk, T. (2011). On the problems of asking for a definition of quality in education. *Scandinavian Journal of Educational Research, 55*(6), 671–684.

www.2020Health.org. (2013). Too Posh to Wash? Reflections on the future of nursing January 2013. Retrieved July 18, 2016, from www.2020health.org/dms/2020health/downloads/reports/2020tooposh_06-02-13

www.educ.cam.ac.uk. (n.d.). *Dialogic teaching and learning*. University of Cambridge Faculty of Education. Retrieved July 19, 2016, from http://www.educ.cam.ac.uk/research/projects/camtalk/dialogic/

Index

A

adult learning, 70, 81–3, 116, 154, 159
adult teaching, 82
apprenticeship models, 8, 71, 73, 74, 103
apprenticeships, 2, 8–10, 73, 74, 102, 141
Approved Education Institution (AEI), 8, 12, 24–6
art and science of nursing, 71, 101, 103, 136

B

Benner, P., 152, 153
Bloom's Taxonomy of Educational Objectives, 63
Bourdieu, P., 111
Briggs Committee, 71, 72
Bruner, J. S., 98, 105, 161, 162

C

Care Quality Commission (CQC), 25, 34, 36
Carper, B. A., 101–4
Cavendish Review, 74
co-created curriculum, 12, 16, 117, 122, 159, 161–5
co-creation, 150, 152, 159, 161, 168, 169
  in nurse education, 121–36, 168
cognitive theory, 76, 97, 128, 161, 168
competency-based education, 62, 78, 124, 152
constructivism, 15, 98, 104–6, 108, 116, 163
contemporary nursing practice, 2, 7, 9, 14, 15, 17, 27, 48, 72, 73, 76, 77, 79, 98, 106, 117, 123, 126, 135, 139–69

© The Author(s) 2018
S. Dyson, *Critical Pedagogy in Nursing*, DOI 10.1057/978-1-137-56891-5

Index

conventional pedagogies, 23, 69, 73–6, 124
co-production
  in education, 109, 110, 124
  in nurse education, 44, 48, 98, 115, 136
Council for Healthcare Regulatory Excellence (CHRE), 25, 26, 140
Council of Deans for Health (CoDH), 2, 4, 9, 26, 27
critical pedagogies, 9, 10, 14, 15, 17, 22, 47, 48, 61, 67, 70, 71, 73, 76–9, 92, 93, 98, 99, 103, 104, 106–8, 116, 133, 154, 155, 159
critical reflection, 83, 85–8, 132–5, 152, 154, 158–61
critical thinking, 2, 14, 23, 26, 27, 63, 76, 89–92, 125, 129, 131, 135, 141, 161, 168
critically reflective learning, 11, 132–4
critically reflective practice, 2, 167
curriculum, 2, 6, 10–12, 24, 61, 70, 72, 80–4, 88–90, 92, 93, 97–101, 105–7, 112, 113, 115–17, 121–3, 125, 127–31, 136, 140, 143–55, 159, 161–8
curriculum development
  in nursing, 2, 11, 16, 22, 47, 84, 93, 105, 115–17, 121, 123, 130, 136, 143–5, 148, 149, 151, 159, 164–6
curriculum models, 11, 145–7, 151, 159, 161, 163

D

Dewey, J., 69, 109, 110, 124
dialogic learning and teaching, 11, 131, 136, 154, 161, 164
dialogic pedagogy, 129–33, 158
dialogic teaching, 130–2
disorientating dilemmas, 85, 86, 157–9

E

English National Board (ENB), 72

F

Francis Inquiry, 2, 7, 8, 10–12, 22, 44, 48, 69, 74, 75, 103, 114, 136, 141
Francis Report, 2, 3, 5, 33, 45, 46, 139
Freire, P., 14, 48, 70, 76, 92, 99, 124, 130, 151, 154, 156, 165
fundamental skills, 93, 153

G

General medical Council (GMC), 44
Giroux, H. A., 14, 61, 70, 76, 107, 124, 154
global health, 13, 14, 48, 53–67
global nurse education, 48, 53–67

H

hidden curriculum, 15, 97, 99–101, 116, 117, 128
higher-order skills, 63
Human Genome Project, 92, 143

Index

I
informal curriculum, 130

M
meaning perspectives, 80, 81, 84, 85, 88, 157–60
Mezirow, J., 70, 80–2, 84–9, 108, 154, 157, 158
Mid Staffordshire NHS Foundation Trust, 1, 6, 13, 22, 26, 33–8, 46, 48, 74, 107, 111, 114
migratory nursing workforce, 49, 53, 64–6
models for cultural competence, 151, 152
modern-day nursing, 45, 130
monitor, 25, 34–8, 91, 92

N
narrative pedagogy, 127–9, 153, 158, 163
National Health Service (NHS), 2, 3, 5, 7, 9, 13, 16, 21, 23, 28–41, 44, 45, 53, 57, 65–7, 74, 80, 92, 93, 103, 104, 108, 114, 122, 142, 150
nurse
    education, 1–6, 8–17, 21–49, 53–67, 69, 72, 80, 97–117, 121, 123, 124, 132, 139–41, 143, 148–51, 153, 155, 161, 164, 166–9
    educationalists, 47, 106, 107
    educators, 2, 5, 6, 9–11, 15–17, 22, 48, 49, 62–4, 67, 69–71, 73, 74, 77, 78, 80, 82–4, 90, 93, 97–100, 104, 106, 107, 111–15, 121, 125, 127–9, 132, 140, 141, 143–5, 148–51, 159, 166, 168
Nurse Educator Core Competencies (NECC), 62
Nursing and Midwifery Council (NMC), 2, 4, 9, 10, 12, 16, 17, 22–7, 44, 47, 64, 65, 67, 69, 70, 72, 74, 77, 78, 84, 93, 98, 106, 115, 121, 127, 135, 136, 139–41, 143–5, 152, 153, 161, 168
nursing compentencies, 75, 79, 116, 136, 162, 168
nursing knowledge, 15, 69, 79, 98, 101–4, 108, 127, 147, 168
nursing pedagogies, 10, 11, 22, 23, 70, 80, 97, 103, 104, 107, 115, 130, 135, 136, 153–5
nursing praxis, 72, 135, 136, 155

O
Office for National Statistics (ONS), 110, 142

P
Pamela Ironside, 124, 153
pedagogies, 2, 9, 11, 12, 14, 15, 17, 22, 23, 47, 48, 61, 67, 69–93, 97–9, 103, 104, 106, 108, 112, 115, 116, 153, 154, 158, 161, 163
personal and moral commitment, 127, 130, 135, 136, 159, 168

praxis, 11, 17, 72, 87, 145, 150–2, 154, 155, 165, 166, 168
process models, 146, 147, 161
product models, 146, 147, 161
Professional Standards Authority (PSA), 26
professionalism, 15, 17, 46, 100, 101, 140
Project 2000, 10, 72, 73

Royal College of Nursing (RCN), 2, 3, 45, 46, 114, 140

social capital, 43, 109–15, 117
spiral curriculum, 15, 98, 105, 106, 162, 168
standards, 4, 5, 9, 10, 21, 22, 24–6, 28, 35, 36, 43, 44, 46–8, 54, 59, 62–4, 67, 69, 70, 72, 77, 84, 93, 98, 100, 107, 127, 135, 145, 152, 161, 166, 167
storytelling, 128, 129, 158, 159
students experiences, 125

Teaching Excellence Framework, 47
The Code for Nurses and Midwives, 44–5

theories and practice in curriculum development, 2, 11, 17, 22, 143–5, 151, 159, 166
theory–practice gap, 10, 15, 75, 97, 98, 100, 116, 164–6
transformative pedagogies, 2, 11, 13, 14, 16, 48, 93, 99, 106, 108, 109, 135, 154, 159, 163, 168, 169

United Kingdom Central Council for Nurses, Midwives and Health Visitors (UKCC), 72

values-based recruitment (VBR), 2, 5, 7, 10
volunteering, 11, 12, 17, 47, 111, 112, 117, 135, 136, 154–8, 160, 163, 164, 167
volunteerism, 135

Willis Commission, 4, 46
World health Organisation (WHO), 14, 54, 57–64, 67, 77